THE HERBAL BODY BOOK

A Natural Approach to Healthier Skin, Hair, and Nails

Stephanie L. Tourles,
Licensed Aesthetician

A Storey Publishing Book

STOREY

Storey Communications, Inc.
Schoolhouse Road
Pownal, Vermont 05261

*The mission of Storey Communications is to serve our customers
by publishing practical information that encourages personal independence
in harmony with the environment.*

Edited by Amanda Haar
Cover design by Carol J. Jessop
Text design and production by Carol J. Jessop
Cover and text illustrations © John Nelson / Represented by Irmeli Holmberg
Line drawing on page 97 by Brigita Fuhrmann
Indexed by Northwind Editorial Services

The information in this book is true and complete to the best of our knowledge. All
recommendations are made without guarantee on the part of the author or Storey
Communications, Inc. The author and the publisher disclaim any liability in connection with the use of this information. For additional information please contact
Storey Communications, Inc., Schoolhouse Road, Pownal, Vermont 05261.

Printed in the United States by R.R. Donnelley
Third Printing, February 1995

Library of Congress Cataloging-in-Publication Data

Tourles, Stephanie L., 1962–
        The herbal body book : a natural approach to healthier hair, skin and nails /
Stephanie L. Tourles.
          p.   cm.
        "A Storey publishing book."
        Includes bibliographical references and index.
        ISBN 0-88266-880-3 : $12.95
        1. Beauty, Personal. 2. Herbal cosmetics. I. Title.
RA778.T64 1994
646.7'2—dc20   94-1481
                                                                        CIP

TABLE OF CONTENTS

For my husband, Bill, who is always there

with his constant love, support, strong self-discipline,

and drive to succeed.

PREFACE

One of the greatest treasures that a woman or a man can have is healthy, radiant skin. A beautiful complexion and glorious body skin are a reflection of our personal life-style practices. The most rigorously followed healthful living plan necessarily includes a nutritious diet, pure water, regular exercise in the fresh air, adequate rest and sleep, sensible stress management, and an effective skin cleansing program. It is this last part, effective skin cleansing, with which this book is intimately concerned.

I am a Licensed Aesthetician in the State of Massachusetts. My specialty is helping individuals achieve their rightful heritage as a "beautiful person," as well as helping them claim their highest health potential through natural procedures.

In my years of experience, I have worked with many commercially prepared products from first-class department stores, as well as with many so-called "natural" products from health food stores. Many of these skin and body cleansers and moisturizers contain highly toxic and irritating ingredients. I have frequently had clients come to me suffering from allergic reactions to these often costly products. Their suffering led me to experiment with totally natural, totally wholesome cosmetic ingredients. My success with this experimentation led to the writing of this book.

By preparing my own facial and body cleansers from fresh herbs, grains, fruits, vegetables, nuts, seeds, and oils, right in my very own kitchen, I have created recipes that produce the desired result of virtually all commercial cosmetics. And with the help and instructions in this book, you too can create natural, health-loving cosmetics that bring a radiance and glow to your face and whole body.

As you're probably aware, commercial cosmetics have one of the highest profit markups of any product on the market. The cost to produce the bottle, label it, and package it is often more than the few cents worth of ingredients in the bottle. In fact, it is not uncommon to pay $20 or more for a two-ounce (60-ml) jar of cream that promises to rejuvenate you by twenty years in twenty days! We all know such a promise can never be kept, but we pay the price anyway because the promise feels so good.

Aside from the obvious savings, creating your own cosmetics at home has many other advantages:

- You have a choice of the purest, freshest, most natural ingredients available. Many of these you probably have in your kitchen cupboard or refrigerator, or can easily purchase them from local health food stores, specialty shops, or mail-order herb companies.

- You can customize natural cosmetics to match your particular skin type or hair condition.

- You can scent your cosmetics with your favorite herbal fragrance.

- By creating your own personal care products, you are contributing to keeping the earth green. Homemade cosmetics contain no toxic chemicals to pollute the earth, they require no animal testing, and the packaging can be recycled.

- In short, nature has truly rewarded us with a multitude of all-natural, wholesome ingredients with which to create a variety of products to both cleanse and nourish your skin, hair, nails, and more.

On the following pages are simple directions for making facial, hair, and body cleansers. You will find chapters offering facial steams, masks, creams, lotions, toners, and hair products, to use and give as gifts. You'll also find a listing of where to buy any unfamiliar ingredients, specifically herbs. In the spirit of realism and economy, beauty and health, I wish you well!

REMEMBER: Nature's Promise . . .
Take care of your skin
and
your skin will reward you with
health and beauty for the rest of your life.

To Your Radiant Health
Stephanie L. Tourles

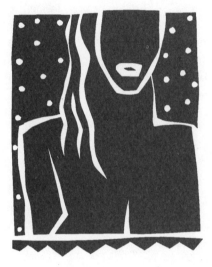

A
Natural
Approach to
Beautiful
Skin

In order to properly care for your skin, it's important that you understand something about its structure and purpose. With this understanding, you'll be better prepared to make decisions about how and why to care for your skin.

YOUR SKIN

The word *system,* according to the *Random House Dictionary,* can be defined as a group or combination of things or parts forming a complex or unified whole. Your skin is a *living system.* Just one square inch consists of approximately 19 million cells, 625 sweat glands, 94 sebaceous glands, 60 hairs, 19,000 sensory nerve cells, 1,250 pain receptors, 13 cold and 78 heat receptors, 160 pressure receptors, and 19 yards of blood vessels.

Your skin serves the body in many capacities, including:

◆ sensory perception
◆ protecting underlying tissues from injury and dehydration
◆ assisting in processes of temperature maintenance and toxic waste elimination
◆ serving as the origination point for the manufacture of vitamin D
◆ giving structure to all organs and systems within the body

To say the least, your skin is an integral part of your living being and one that plays a vital role within your body's supportive and functional capacities. It's essential that you learn how to care for it and nourish it so that it will remain healthy regardless of the climate you live in or your chronological age.

Contrary to popular opinion, beautiful skin doesn't come in pretty bottles filled with a vitamin/hormone cream that smells of artificial fragrance. Nor does it come from chemicals designed to dry up acne pimples, such as tetracycline, Accutane, or benzoyl peroxide. Truly beautiful skin comes as a result of adhering to a program of feeding your body a proper diet, getting daily exercise and adequate sleep, and by employing an appropriate cleansing regime.

Though this book is primarily concerned with natural skin care through the use of wholesome products, I want to stress the importance of a proper diet and daily exercise in maintaining beautiful skin.

Diet

The skin is one of the first organs of the body to be affected by poor diet, vitamin and mineral deficiencies, and improper elimination. Moist, clear, radiant skin is generally a sign of good health, while skin that is dry and flaky or oily and pimply can be indicative of internal problems, especially where nutrition is concerned.

Your diet should consist of foods that are high in complex carbohydrates, low in fat, high in fiber, and moderate in protein. A wide variety of foods in their whole, natural state should be consumed daily, including several servings each of fresh and dried fruits, vegetables, whole grains, plus a few fresh nuts and seeds. If you consume dairy products, they should be non-fat, and cheeses should be eaten in moderation because of their high fat content. Meat eaters should try to limit their meat consumption to three to four ounces (85 to 133 g) per day (about the size of a deck of cards) and try to buy only free-range chickens, fresh, deep-sea fish, and extremely lean beef that was raised without hormones and antibiotics. Of course, it goes without saying, one should eliminate smoking and consume alcohol in small amounts, if at all.

According to Drs. Robert and Elizabeth McCarter, contributing authors of *The Life Science Health System,* "A healthy skin sings of a well-nourished body, of systemic equilibrium, of balance, of homeostasis, of sound living practices, of good inheritance, of vitality, of a clean, free-flowing unobstructed blood stream, and of organs functioning silently and efficiently in a body at peace."

A wholesome, balanced diet such as this nourishes the inner body and is reflected on the outer body as gorgeous skin. As you plan your daily or weekly menus, try to remember that your skin is the visible evidence of the condition of your inner health. It is the mirror that reflects your present state of health or ill-health.

Exercise

Daily exercise is vital to your physical well-being, and can help your mental health as well by eliminating or reducing stress. By taking a brisk 30-minute walk and performing approximately 15 minutes of gentle stretches each and every day, you stimulate your metabolism, keep your muscles and joints loose and flexible, enjoy a bit of fresh air and sunshine, and get your heart pumping and blood flowing. Try to exercise vigorously enough so that you work up a good sweat. Sweating cools your skin and eliminates waste through your pores.

If you don't like to walk, choose whatever you enjoy: biking, jogging, swimming, aerobic classes, tennis, or even roller blading. There really is something for everyone. It's up to you to find it and stick with it.

If you are over the age of thirty-five, have been inactive for a period of time, or have any health problems, be sure to get your doctor's okay *before* beginning any exercise program. For further information on diet and exercise, see the *Appendix* for reading suggestions.

CARING FOR YOUR SKIN

To keep your skin deep-down clean, no matter whether it's oily, combination, normal, or dry, all that is necessary is that you observe these five basic practices: cleansing, toning (sometimes referred to as clarifying or freshening), moisturizing, high water intake, and dry brushing.

The first three should be performed as a series of steps. Here's how:

1. Cleansing: This step, I feel, is the most important. Twice a day, using a washcloth or facial sponge, apply the appropriate facial cleanser for your skin type to your face and throat and massage gently, using upward, circular strokes. This step should take about a minute. Now, rinse your face with clean, warm water to remove all traces of the cleanser and pat dry.

Never, never, never *scrub* your facial skin! I've actually seen some women scrub their face so hard you'd think they were trying to clean their kitchen sink! Always be gentle. Now, on to the next step.

2. Toning: A toner or astringent is designed to remove any traces of cleanser that have been left behind during the cleansing process and to restore the skin to its normally acid pH. To apply your toner, simply saturate a 100% cotton ball with your chosen herbal liquid and apply to your face and throat using gentle, upward strokes. Do not pat dry. You will want to lock in this precious moisture by performing the next step.

3. Moisturizing: Using a moisturizer should become a part of everyone's daily routine regardless of whether you think your skin is too oily to benefit from one or not. A moisturizer is designed to prevent dehydration (loss of water) from occurring in your skin. Your skin can be extremely oily, but also suffer from a lack of water. A good moisturizer serves as a barrier between your skin and the environment. It will help to keep your skin younger-looking longer.

To benefit from all that a moisturizer has to offer, simply apply the appropriate moisturizer to your already moist face and throat, using upward, circular strokes until the moisturizer disappears. You're finished!

These three steps should take you no longer than five minutes, twice a day — a small amount of time to devote daily for a lifetime of beautiful skin!

Finally, let me mention the two last secrets for beautiful skin: drinking pure, clean water and dry brushing.

4. Drink plenty of Water: Whether in the form of raw fruits and vegetables or several glasses of plain water, sufficient water consumption is essential to maintaining soft, moist, glowing skin. Any model will tell you that he or she drinks a minimum of six glasses a day. I personally enjoy four to six glasses, plus consuming a high water content diet.

For those of you who just hate plain water, try adding a squeeze of lime, lemon, or orange juice. This will turn your plain, blah water into a very refreshing drink. A splash of cranberry juice tastes great too!

TAKING THE MYSTERY OUT OF pH

You've seen it on everything from shampoos to soap, but what exactly is pH? The pH (potential hydrogen) of a liquid refers to its degree of acidity or alkalinity. Meters and indicator papers have been developed for the measurement of pH. The pH scale goes from 0 to 14, with the neutral point being 7. Anything below a 7 on the pH scale is regarded as acid. The lower the pH, the greater the degree of acidity. Anything above a 7 is regarded as alkaline. The higher the pH, the greater is the degree of alkalinity. The pH of normal, healthy skin ranges from 4.5 to 6 and is most often referred to as 5.5. Your skin maintains its proper pH level by forming an acid mantle on its surface from the combined secretions of your sweat and oil glands. By using a toner to keep your skin at its proper pH level, you help prevent bacterial penetration (which occurs when skin is too acidic) and flaking and scaling because of moisture loss (which occurs when skin is too alkaline).

Regardless of your skin type, you should always look for a toner with a pH level in the range of 4.5 to 6.

5. Dry Brushing: Dry brushing is a *must* for smooth, clear skin. Over the course of a day your skin eliminates more than a pound of waste through thousands of tiny sweat glands. In fact, about one-third of all the body's impurities are excreted this way. But, if your pores are clogged by tight-fitting clothes, aluminum-containing antiperspirants, and mineral oil-based moisturizers, there's no way for these toxic by-products to escape. Over time, these cells build up and eventually you will get sick because the toxins have to seek another route to escape from your body. Not to mention that your skin will begin to look pale, pasty, and pimply. There is a solution...dry brushing.

Dry brushing is performed on dry skin — not oiled, not damp, but dry before you shower. Using a natural-fiber brush the size of your palm, preferably with a handle, you simply brush your entire body — except your face (and breasts, if you're a woman) — for 5 to 10 minutes. Daily. Do not brush hard. You will have to start *very gently* and work your way up to more vigorous brushing, but never scrub. It will take your skin awhile to get used to this new treatment. Begin brushing your hands first, in between the fingers, then arms, under-arms, neck, chest, stomach, back, then on to each leg beginning with the feet. You will feel wonderfully invigorated when finished, and your skill will glow! Then, just jump in the shower, bathe as you usually do, and all of the dead skin you just exfoliated is washed away. Be sure to pat, not rub, your skin dry, and apply a light moisturizer after you shower.

A DRY BRUSH BONUS

Here's an added plus to dry brushing...because dry-brushing opens your clogged pores and aids in elimination, your cellulite will begin to diminish. Trust me...it works. Follow a good, low-fat diet and exercise program, and it will work even faster.

It's a good idea to wash your brush with soap and water every week or so to keep it free of skin debris.

For more in-depth reading on dry-brushing, see the *Appendix* .

"Not only does beauty fade, but it leaves a record upon the face as to what became of it."   — Elbert Hubbard

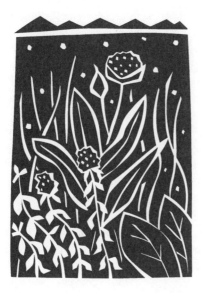

The Natural
Qualities
of Herbs
and Other
Ingredients

CHAPTER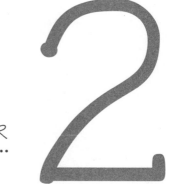

This chapter details the ingredients called for in the personal care recipes that begin in chapter 4. I've also listed many other herbs and nonherbal items which can be used as substitutes when the item called for in a particular recipe is unavailable.

Where do you find these ingredients? Your local health food store is the first place to check for beeswax, lanolin, cocoa butter, essential and vegetable oils, seeds, and grains. If you have no luck, or there's no health food store nearby, try the local pharmacy or cosmetic supply house. The Yellow Pages are also an excellent place to look for ingredients. Look under such headings as Botanicals, Herbs, Nurseries / Garden Centers, Health/Natural Food Stores, Perfumes, Pharmacies, Spices, or Oils. If you have a green thumb and enjoy gardening, you can grow many of the herbs from seed or plants bought at your local garden center. Or you can forage for herbs in the wild. If you decide to go this route, be sure to purchase a good illustrated herb book (preferably with color pictures) and educate yourself while you go hiking through the woods and meadows.

For a detailed listing of mail order herb companies, cosmetic supplies, and natural food companies, see *Appendix*.

A WORD ABOUT OILS

Many of the recipes in this book call for oils such as grapeseed oil or sweet almond oil. When purchasing these oils, look for the "cold-pressed" version. Although more expensive than refined oils found in supermarkets that contain petroleum residues from the solvents used in the extraction process, cold-pressed oils are 100% pure and contain more of the fruit, vegetable, nut, or plant's natural ingredients. Cold-pressed oils are better for your skin and the environment.

DRYING YOUR OWN HERBS

You may be surprised by how easy it is to dry many of the herbs from your garden. No matter which tecnhique you choose, it is best to dry your herbs as soon as they are picked so that none of their beneficial properties are lost. Other points to keep in mind include:

◆ Try to harvest your herbs as soon as they come into bloom.
◆ Using a sharp knife, gather herbs in the early to mid-morning after any evening dew has had a chance to dry but before the sun becomes too hot.
◆ Be careful to harvest herbs that are free of insects, disease, and have not been treated with pesticides. Your herbs should be relatively dirt-free but if they are dusty or if you have gathered them from a roadside where they have been exposed to exhaust, you can quickly rinse them in cool water and immediately pat dry with a paper towel. Be sure to pat gently as the leaves will bruise easily.
◆ Avoid overdrying as it can diminish the valuable properties of the herb.
◆ Dried herbs should be stored in a cool, moisture-free place away from direct sunlight.

Drying by Hanging

To dry your herbs by hanging, simply gather five stems of a single herb together in a bundle. Secure the stems together using a string, rubber bands, or clothes pins. Bundles should be hung upside down in a well-ventilated, dimly lit area. The ideal temperature for drying is between 65°F (20°C) and 80°F (25°C). Leave plenty of room between bundles to ensure good air circulation and to keep scents from mingling. As many herbs look similar when dried, you may find it helpful to label your bundles.

Herbs can take anywhere from four days to three weeks to dry. Leaves should be brittle but not so dry as to easily shatter. Flower petals should feel dry and crisp.

Drying on Screens

Many herbs can also be successfully dried on wire screens or tightly stretched netting. The open mesh of the screen or net allows air to flow freely around the herb and quickly evaporate the plants' moisture.

To prepare herbs for screen drying, separate the leaves and flower petals from the stem and spread in a single layer over the screen. Leave enough space between leaves and petals to allow for good air circulation. Drying times will vary between four days and three weeks.

ALMOND, MEAL *(Prunus amygdalus)*
Parts Used: Raw almonds, ground into a meal
Cosmetic Properties: Emollient, bleaching, exfoliant
Possible Substitutes: Sunflower seed meal
Where to Find: Health food store, mail order

ALMOND OIL, SWEET *(Prunus amygdalus)*
Cosmetic Properties: Removes eye makeup, emollient, all-purpose body oil
Possible Substitutes: Cold-pressed apricot, avocado, or sunflower oil
Where to Find: Health food store, mail order

ALOE *(Aloe vera or A. barbadensis)*
Parts Used: Gel from leaves. Fresh is preferred.
Cosmetic Properties: Astringent for normal-to-oily skin, relieves sunburn, minor skin burns, insect bites. Helps restore natural pH level to skin
Where to Find: Plant is available from nurseries or garden centers. Bottled juice available from health food store and mail order.

APPLE CIDER VINEGAR
Cosmetic Properties: Astringent (diluted with water), soothing, relieves itchy, dry, scaly skin. Restores natural pH level to skin.
Where to Find: Health food store, mail order, or grocery store

APRICOT OIL *(Prunus armeniaca)*
Parts Used: Oil from kernel
Cosmetic Properties: Emollient. Excellent for softening the delicate skin around the eye and on the throat. This light oil is also good for removing all types of makeup.
Possible Substitutes: Grapeseed oil
Where to Find: Health food store, mail order

ARROWROOT *(Maranta arundinacea)*
Parts Used: Powdered rhizomes
Cosmetic Properties: A bland, gentle powder often used in making herbal body powders
Possible Substitutes: Cornstarch
Where to Find: Health food store, mail order

AVOCADO OIL *(Persea americana)*
Parts Used: Pulp, oil

Cosmetic Properties: The pulp is very fatty. Both oil and pulp are quite nourishing and conditioning for dry skin and hair.
Possible Substitutes: Sweet almond, castor, or jojoba oils
Where to Find: Health food store, mail order

BAKING SODA
Common Name: Sodium bicarbonate
Cosmetic Properties: Very alkaline with skin soothing and softening properties. Relieves bee stings and the itching from rashes. Deodorizes feet and underarms. Softens bath water.
Where to Find: Grocery store

BASIL *(Ocimum basilicum)*
Common Name: Sweet basil
Parts Used: Essential oil
Cosmetic Properties: Conditioning, reported to stimulate hair growth, fragrant
Possible Substitute: Essential oil of rosemary is much less expensive and almost as effective as basil.
Where to Find: Health food store, mail order

BENZOIN GUM *(Styrax benzoin)*
Common Name: Gum Benjamin
Parts Used: Gum, tincture of benzoin
Cosmetic Properties: Mild antiseptic, fixative in potpourri and body powders, preservative
Where to Find: Health food store, mail order

BLACKBERRY *(Rubus villosus)*
Parts Used: Leaves
Cosmetic Properties: Astringent, cleansing
Possible Substitutes: Burdock, strawberry, sage, raspberry
Where to Find: Health food store, mail order, growing wild, grow your own

BORAX
Common Name: Sodium borate
Parts Used: White, crystalline mineral powder
Cosmetic Properties: It is used mainly as a water softener and emulsifier in natural cosmetics. Also a weak antiseptic.
Where to Find: Health food store, mail order, pharmacy. You can use the borax found in the clothes detergent section of your grocery store.

BURDOCK *(Arctium lappa)*
Common Names: Beggar's buttons, burr seed, cocklebur
Parts Used: Leaves and crushed seeds
Cosmetic Properties: Cleansing, astringent
Possible Substitutes: Strawberry or raspberry leaves
Where to Find: Health food store, mail order, growing wild

CALENDULA *(Calendula officinalis)*
Common Name: Pot marigold. Calendula or pot marigold is often called simply "marigold." *Do not,* however, confuse calendula with the African marigold (botanical name: *tagetes)* which is commonly planted in flower and vegetable gardens. While an attractive and bug-repelling addition to the garden, the African marigold is *not* a medicinal herb.
Parts Used: Flower petals, tincture (an alcohol-based herbal extract), fresh juice from petals
Cosmetic Properties: Healing, hair coloring for red or blond hair. Good when used as the main herbal ingredient in a cream or salve to be applied to irritated, rashy, or chapped skin.
Where to Find: Health food store, mail order, grow your own

CARROT SEED, ESSENTIAL OIL *(Daucus carota)*
Parts Used: Essential oil
Cosmetic Properties: Excellent for sensitive skin. Tones and stimulates elasticity. The oil can be mixed with a carrier oil, such as sweet almond or jojoba, and used to cleanse the skin or as an under-eye moisturizing treatment.
Where to Find: Health food store, mail order

CASTILE SOAP
Parts Used: Liquid or soap cake
Cosmetic Properties: A gentle, olive oil-based soap that can be used to bathe the entire body and used as a base in herbal shampoos
Where to Find: Health food store, mail order, and some grocery stores

CASTOR BEAN *(Ricinus communis)*
Common Names: Castor oil plant, palma Christi
Parts Used: Oil
Cosmetic Properties: Thick and emollient. Makes hair shiny when used as a conditioner. Good for dry skin and brittle nails.
Where to Find: Health food store, mail order, better drug and grocery stores

CHAMOMILE, GERMAN *(Matricaria chamomilla)*

Parts Used: Flowers, essential oil

Cosmetic Properties: Anti-inflammatory, healing, mild astringent, fragrant. Lightens and brightens blond hair.

Where to Find: Health food store, mail order, or grow your own

CHICKWEED *(Stellaria media)*

Common Name: Indian chickweed, satin flower

Parts Used: Leaves

Cosmetic Properties: Soothing to irritated skin

Possible Substitutes: Comfrey leaves

Where to Find: Health food store, mail order, growing wild

CLARY SAGE *(Salvia sclarea)*

Common Name: French sage

Parts Used: Leaves, essential oil

Cosmetic Properties: Mainly used in perfumery. Makes a relaxing bath. Makes a good hair conditioner. Mild astringent.

Where to Find: Health food store, mail order

COCOA OR CACAO BUTTER *(Theobroma cacao)*

Parts Used: Cocoa butter

Cosmetic Properties: Emollient. Cocoa butter is hard at room temperature, but melts when applied to the skin. It also smells like chocolate!

Where to Find: Health food store, mail order, better drug stores

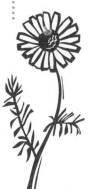

COCONUT OIL *(Cocos nucifera)*

Parts Used: Oil

Cosmetic Properties: Emollient. This oil becomes hard at room temperature, and like cocoa butter, melts at body temperature. It is a good oil for all-over use. Some people swear by coconut oil as the ultimate skin softener, hair conditioner, and after-sun treatment.

Where to Find: Health food store, mail order

COMFREY *(Symphytum officinale)*

Common Names: Gum plant, knitback, healing herb

Parts Used: Leaves, roots

Cosmetic Properties: Soothing, healing, mild astringent, emollient

Where to Find: Health food store, mail order, growing wild, grow your own

CORNMEAL *(Zea mays)*
Common Name: Indian corn
Parts Used: White or yellow corn, ground into meal
Cosmetic Properties: Exfoliant
Where to Find: Health food store, mail order, grocery store

CREAM, HEAVY DAIRY
Cosmetic Properties: Fatty and emollient. Super for dry skin when mixed with facial and body scrub mixtures to make a paste.
Possible Substitutes: Whole milk
Where to Find: Grocery store

CUCUMBER *(Cucumis sativus)*
Parts Used: Strained pulp, juice
Cosmetic Properties: Mildly astringent, soothing, has a slight bleaching action which aids in removing dead skin cells
Where to Find: Grocery store, grow your own

ELDER FLOWER *(Sambucus canadensis)*
Common Names: Elderberry, American elder, black elder
Parts Used: Flowers
Cosmetic Properties: Healing, very gentle astringent, antiseptic, softening, fragrant
Possible Substitute: Comfrey
Where to Find: Health food store, mail order, growing wild, grow your own

EPSOM SALT
Common Name: Magnesium sulfate
Cosmetic Properties: Relieves aches and pains. Good for tired feet when used in a foot bath.
Where to Find: Grocery and drug stores

EUCALYPTUS *(Eucalyptus globulus)*
Common Name: Blue gum
Parts Used: Essential oil
Cosmetic Properties: Antiseptic, cooling, fragrant. Makes a good wash for wounds and, when mixed with a carrier oil, makes a good liniment for sore muscles.
Possible Substitutes: Peppermint, spearmint
Where to Find: Health food store, mail order

FENNEL *(Foeniculum vulgare)*

Parts Used: Seeds

Cosmetic Properties: Cleansing, soothing to irritated skin, fragrant

Where to Find: Health food store, growing wild, grow your own

FRENCH CLAY

Cosmetic Properties: Tightening, absorbs oil from skin

Possible Substitutes: Kaolin (China clay) or bentonite (clay found in the midwest U.S. and Canada)

Where to Find: Health food store, mail order

FULLER'S EARTH

Common Name: Diatomaceous earth. This substance looks and acts almost like clay, but the two are made of different materials. Fuller's earth is a relatively pure form of silica. Clay consists of silica, aluminum, magnesium, calcium, iron, titanium, phosphorus, sodium, and potassium. They are *not* interchangeable.

Cosmetic Properties: Basically the same as French clay

Possible Substitutes: French clay is preferred over Fuller's earth

Where to Find: Health food store, mail order

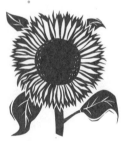

GERANIUM *(Pelargonium)*

Common Name: Scented geranium

Parts Used: Leaves, essential oil

Cosmetic Properties: Mild astringent, fragrant

Where to Find: Health food store, mail order, grow your own

GLYCERIN

Cosmetic Properties: Emollient. Found in animal and vegetable fats. It acts as a humectant, which means it draws moisture from the air to the skin. Great for chapped skin.

Where to Find: Health food store, mail order, better drug stores

GRAPESEED OIL

Cosmetic Properties: Emollient, nonallergenic. One of the best oils for making massage and bath oils because it is light and nongreasy. Like apricot oil, it is good for mature skin and delicate eye and throat areas.

Where to Find: Health food store, mail order

HONEY
Cosmetic Properties: Emollient, humectant, soothing
Where to Find: Health food store, grocery store, mail order, apiary

JASMINE *(Jasminum officinale)*
Parts Used: Flowers, essential oil
Cosmetic Properties: Has a calming, sensual fragrance. Extremely expensive. Cleanses and soothes the skin. Used in many floral perfumes.
Where to Find: Health food store, mail order, grow your own

JOJOBA *(Simmondsis chinensis)*
Parts Used: Oil, very expensive
Cosmetic Properties: Excellent conditioner for hair, scalp, skin, and nails. Wonderful all-purpose skin lubricant. Jojoba oil is very similar to our own sebum, the natural moisturizing oils secreted by the skin. I like to use it because it does not go rancid like other oils and requires no refrigeration.
Possible Substitutes: Sweet almond oil, though not as good and must be refrigerated
Where to Find: Health food store, mail order

JUNIPER *(Juniperus communis)*
Parts Used: Essential oil, berries
Cosmetic Properties: Antiseptic, fragrant. Good for tired, aching feet, cooling and refreshing.
Possible Substitutes: Eucalyptus, peppermint
Where to Find: Health food store, mail order, grow your own

LADY'S MANTLE *(Alchemilla vulgaris)*
Parts Used: Leaves
Cosmetic Properties: Healing, soothing. Makes a good astringent for normal-to-dry and sensitive skin.
Possible Substitutes: Orange flowers, calendula
Where to Find: Health food store, mail order, growing wild, grow your own

LANOLIN, anhydrous
Common Names: Wool fat or wax
Cosmetic Properties: Emollient, holds water on the skin. Because it contains less than 0.25% water, anhydrous lanolin can absorb water and it acts as a great emulsifier for creams and lotions.
Where to Find: Health food store, mail order

LAVENDER *(Lavandula vera* or *L. officinalis)*
Parts Used: Flowers, essential oil
Cosmetic Properties: Hair conditioner, fragrant, antiseptic, soothing to skin
Possible Substitutes: Rosemary, though more astringent. Can be mixed with comfrey.
Where to Find: Health food store, mail order, grow your own

LEMON *(Citrus limon)*
Parts Used: Juice, essential oil, rind
Cosmetic Properties: Strong astringent, fragrant, invigorating, disinfectant, bleaching to skin and hair, helps restore natural pH level to skin. Put elbows in scooped out lemon halves to soften and lighten rough, dark skin.
Possible Substitutes: Tangerine, for the astringent property
Where to Find: Grocery store, grow your own

LEMON BALM *(Melissa officinalis)*
Common Names: Melissa, balm mint
Parts Used: Leaves, essential oil
Cosmetic Properties: Cleansing and antiseptic, fragrant
Possible Substitutes: Peppermint, lemongrass
Where to Find: Health food store, mail order, growing wild, grow your own

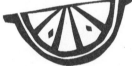

LEMONGRASS *(Cymbopogon citratus)*
Parts Used: Leaves, essential oil
Cosmetic Properties: Cleanser for dry and oily skin; it is reported to normalize oil production. Fragrant, antiseptic.
Where to Find: Health food store, mail order

MARSHMALLOW *(Althaea officinalis)*
Parts Used: Root, dried
Cosmetic Properties: Emollient, softening, soothing. When the dried roots are boiled in water, they produce a gummy substance or mucilage which is good for inflamed skin, dry hands, or sunburn.
Possible Substitutes: Comfrey roots
Where to Find: Health food store, mail order

MUSK OIL (synthetic)
Cosmetic Properties: Fragrant oil used for perfume and in massage and bath oils
Where to Find: Health food store, mail order

MYRRH (Commiphora myrrha)
Common Name: Gum myrrh tree
Parts Used: Resin, tincture of myrrh
Cosmetic Properties: Antiseptic, astringent, disinfectant. Good for sore throat, teeth, gums, and bad breath. Also acts as preservative.
Where to Find: Health food store, mail order

NETTLE (Urtica dioica)
Common Names: Stinging nettle, common nettle
Parts Used: Leaves
Cosmetic Properties: Slightly astringent, improves circulation, hair conditioner, stimulates hair growth
Where to Find: Health food store, mail order, growing wild

NON-PETROLEUM JELLY
Cosmetic Properties: Soothing to rough, dry, chapped skin. It is made from plant-based waxes and oils as opposed to petroleum.
Where to Find: Health food store, mail order

OATS (Avena sativa)
Parts Used: Oatmeal, ground into a fine flourlike meal
Cosmetic Properties: Soothing to irritated skin. Makes a good base for facial scrubs and masks. Colloidal oatmeal is ground extremely fine and is great for relieving the itch caused by poison ivy and oak. Also good for rashy, dry, sensitive skin.
Where to Find: Health food store, mail order, grocery, or drug store

OLIVE OIL (Olea europaea)
Parts Used: Oil. Virgin olive oil is preferred.
Cosmetic Properties: Emollient. Can be used in a pinch when other oils are unavailable
Possible Substitutes: Cold-pressed avocado, apricot, or sunflower oil
Where to Find: Health food store, grocery store

ORANGE (Citrus sinensis)
Parts Used: Flowers
Cosmetic Properties: Emollient and soothing when used in facial steams. A mixture of orange flower water and glycerin makes a good toner for dry, sensitive skin, and for individuals with broken capillaries.
Possible Substitute: Elder Flower
Where to Find: Health food store, mail order

PAPAYA *(Carica papaya)*
Parts Used: Strained pulp
Cosmetic Properties: Contains a protein-digesting enzyme (papain), which helps dissolve the dead outer layer of skin, revealing the soft, fresh, new layer underneath. Also, helps restore the skin's natural pH level.
Where to Find: Grocery store

PARSLEY *(Petroselinum sativum)*
Common Names: Garden parsley, rock parsley
Parts Used: Leaves
Cosmetic Properties: Soothing and healing for those who suffer with bad cases of acne, eczema, and psoriasis. Can be chewed to sweeten breath. Also makes a good rinse for all hair types.
Where to Find: Health food store, mail order, most grocery stores, grow your own

PATCHOULI *(Pogostemon cablin)*
Parts Used: Leaves, essential oil
Cosmetic Properties: The oil is used mainly in perfumes as the main scent or as a blender with other scents. The herb and oil can be used to freshen musty rooms.
Where to Find: Health food store, mail order

PEACH *(Prunus persica)*
Parts Used: Pulp of fruit
Cosmetic Properties: Enriching, moisturizing, and lightly toning
Where to Find: Grocery store

PEPPERMINT *(Mentha piperita)*
Parts Used: Leaves, essential oil
Cosmetic Properties: Mild astringent, cooling and refreshing, fragrant, antiseptic. Can be used as a breath freshener and mouthwash.
Possible Substitutes: Spearmint (though not as strong)
Where to Find: Health food store, mail order, growing wild, grow your own

PINE *(many different species)*
Parts Used: Needles, essential oil
Cosmetic Properties: Stimulating to the senses and soothing to the skin. Fragrant.
Where to Find: Health food store, mail order, growing wild

PINEAPPLE *(Ananas comosus)*
Parts Used: Strained pulp, juice
Cosmetic Properties: Slight bleaching action, astringent
Where to Find: Grocery store. Be sure to buy a ripe pineapple since they do not ripen much after they are picked.

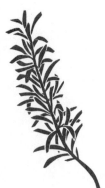

QUASSIA *(Picraena excelsa)*
Common Names: Bitter ash or bitter wood
Parts Used: Wood chips
Cosmetic Properties: Chips are simmered in water to make a brightening rinse for dark hair. Best used on normal or oily hair because of astringent qualities. Good for those with dandruff.
Where to Find: Health food store, mail order

RASPBERRY *(Rubus idaeus)*
Common Name: Garden raspberry
Parts Used: Leaves, fruit
Cosmetic Properties: Astringent, good for rashes and sores
Possible Substitutes: Strawberry, blackberry
Where to Find: Health food store, mail order, growing wild, grow your own

RHUBARB *(Rheum palmatum)*
Parts Used: Roots, crushed and dried
Cosmetic Properties: Astringent. Crushed roots are simmered and the resulting liquid is poured through light brown or blonde hair to brighten and bring out blonde highlights.
Where to Find: Grocery store, grow your own

ROSE *(Rosa)* species
Common Name: Red garden rose
Parts Used: Petals, essential oil
Cosmetic Properties: Mild astringent for dry or chapped skin, helps restore pH. Excellent when mixed with glycerin as a dry skin wash and skin freshener.
Where to Find: Health food store, mail order, grow your own

ROSEMARY *(Rosemarinus officinalis)*
Parts Used: Leaves, essential oil
Cosmetic Properties: Mild astringent, healing, darkens and conditions hair, stimulates hair growth, stimulating to senses, fragrant. Good for aching muscles when used in the bath. Excellent when

mixed with essential oils of lavender and basil as a hair and scalp conditioner.

Where to Find: Health food store, mail order, grow your own

ROSEWATER

Cosmetic Properties: Very mild astringent. Makes a great cleanser for dry skin when mixed 50/50 with glycerin.

Where to Find: Health food store, mail order

SAGE *(Salvia officinalis)*

Common Names: Garden sage, Spanish sage

Parts Used: Leaves

Cosmetic Properties: Astringent, darkens hair, antiseptic, fragrant, strong disinfectant

Possible Substitutes: May be mixed with rosemary or lavender or a combination of both

Where to Find: Health food store, mail order, grow your own

SANDALWOOD *(Santalum album)*

Parts Used: Essential oil

Cosmetic Properties: Disinfectant, fragrant. Great for dry skin and hair.

Where to Find: Health food store, mail order

SEA SALT

Cosmetic Properties: Healing to open sores and pimples. Can be used in a body scrub mixture or a soothing foot bath.

Possible Substitutes: Table salt (can be irritating to those with sensitive skin)

Where to Find: Health food store or mail order

STRAWBERRY (WILD) *(Fragaria vesca)*

Common Names: Mountain strawberry, snake berry

Parts Used: Leaves, fruit

Cosmetic Properties: Mild astringent, soothing. The berry can be used to freshen the breath and whiten the teeth. Both the leaves and berry juice make a good wash for oily skin.

Where to Find: Health food store, mail order, growing wild, grow your own

SUNFLOWER SEED MEAL *(Helianthus annuus)*

Parts Used: Fresh raw, hulled seeds, ground into a fine meal

Cosmetic Properties: Emollient, exfoliant

Where to Find: Health food store, mail order, grocery store, or grow your own. When you purchase hulled sunflower seeds, make sure they do not have any black or brown spots indicating rancidity on them. Purchase seeds from a reputable dealer, preferably one who refrigerates seeds, and be sure to refrigerate or freeze your seeds at home.

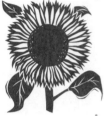

TEA TREE *(Melaleuca alternifolia)*
Parts Used: Essential oil
Cosmetic Properties: Healing, antiseptic, germicidal, astrigent
Where to Find: Health food store, mail order

VETIVERT *(Vetiveria zizanioides)*
Parts Used: Essential oil
Cosmetic Properties: Aids in cleansing and soothing dry skin. Mixes well with essential oil of sandalwood and patchouli as fragrance oil.
Where to Find: Health food store, mail order

VITAMIN A
Common Names: Vitamin A can come from a number of natural sources such as: lemongrass, fish liver oil, and beta carotene.
Parts Used: Use capsule form, measured in international units (IU).
Cosmetic Properties: Vitamin A is healing and soothing for all skin types, especially rough, dry, or blemished skin.
Where to Find: Health food store, mail order. Rarely will high-quality vitamin A be sold in grocery stores.

VITAMIN E
Common Names: Use only 100% natural d-alpha tocopherol from mixed tocopherols (refer to jar label). All other forms are synthetic.
Parts Used: Use capsule form, measured in international units (IU).
Cosmetic Properties: Acts as preservative when added to other oils or cosmetics. Prevents rancidity. Aids in the prevention of scar tissue resulting from burns, cuts, and sores. Reported to slow the aging process. Excellent for all skin types.
Where to Find: Health food store, mail order. Rarely will the natural form of vitamin E be found in grocery stores.

WALNUT, BLACK *(Juglans nigra)*
Parts Used: Nut hulls
Cosmetic Properties: Very astringent. When hulls are simmered

in water, they produce a very dark brown liquid that can be used to brighten black or brunette hair. The same infusion will darken light-colored hair.

Where to Find: Health food store, mail order, growing wild

WHEAT GERM

Parts Used: Raw, fresh wheat germ, wheat germ oil

Cosmetic Properties: Raw, fresh wheat germ is the heart of wheat kernel. It is rich in protein, vitamin B1, and in soluble dietary fiber. The oil in particular is one of the richest sources of vitamin E. Both are excellent for normal and dry skin.

Where to Find: Health food store, mail order. Make sure it is very fresh and store in the refrigerator to avoid rancidity.

WITCH HAZEL *(Hamamelis virginiana)*

Parts Used: Bark, leaves

Cosmetic Properties: Mild astringent, cleansing

Where to Find: Health food store, mail order, growing wild. Most grocery and drug stores carry the bottled version.

YARROW *(Achillea millefolium)*

Common Name: Milfoil

Parts Used: Leaves

Cosmetic Properties: Excellent astringent, douche, cleansing, healing

Where to Find: Health food store, mail order, growing wild, grow your own

YLANG-YLANG *(Cananga odorata)*

Parts Used: Essential oil

Cosmetic Properties: Sweet smelling floral oil used in perfume oils and in massage. The scent is said to lift spirits and stimulate sexual energy. Can be expensive.

Where to Find: Health food store, mail order

YOGURT, plain

Cosmetic Properties: Mild astringent, slight bleaching action. Evens out skin tone when used as a mask.

Possible Substitutes: Lemon juice, cut with water 50% to reduce acidity

Where to Find: Grocery store

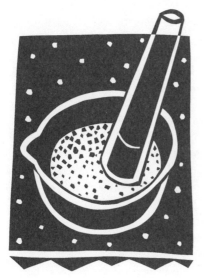

Getting
Ready to
Make and Use
Your Own
Cosmetics

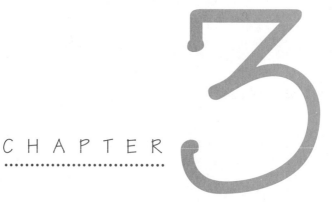

CHAPTER

Making your own personal care products from natural ingredients is easy and can be a lot of fun. Only basic kitchen equipment and cooking skills are necessary for producing wonderfully fresh, body-nurturing creations.

Two equipment lists follow. The first includes equipment needed for preparing your cosmetics, and the second, storage container options identified by which work best with the particular cosmetic you've just prepared.

And finally, a list of applicators and cleansing tools identifies some common and not so common items that will ensure you get the most from your creations.

FOR PREPARING

Blender. This is great for whipping creams and lotions in quantities of one cup (237 ml) or more. When mixing smaller quantities, I find it difficult to get all the cream or lotion out of the bottom of the blender. A blender can also be used to grind oatmeal, almonds, and sunflower seeds for facial and body scrubs, but a food processor or nut/seed grinder usually works *much* better.

Bowls. You'll need various sizes in glass, enamel, or stainless steel. I use small bowls for mixing masks, single-serving facial scrubs, and dentifrices, and larger bowls for mixing the herbs in herbal facial steams and body powders. I sometimes use plastic bowls for mixing. Don't use them if you've stored tomato sauce or anything strongly flavored in them before, since plastic tends to absorb odors and flavors and can leach them into your cosmetics.

Cheesecloth. Used for straining herbs from liquids and for making bath and wash bags. Panty hose or coarsely woven burlap make good substitutes.

Double Boiler. This consists of one pan set inside another of the same size. The bottom pan is filled with water that is allowed to boil, thus heating the top pan. I occasionally use a double boiler to melt wax, cocoa butter, or coconut oil, and to warm oils when making various creams, lotions, and lip balms. The advantage of a double boiler is that it produces a gentle, even heat. Also, it is impossible to scorch your ingredients if you happen to get called away from the kitchen. Usually, though, I simply choose a basic stainless steel pan (or pans), and use the lowest setting on my stove to melt and warm my ingredients, stirring occasionally.

Eyedropper (glass). Used for measuring drops of essential oil and tincture of benzoin. Glass is preferable as it does not retain the scent from the previous ingredient as plastic does. Rinse dropper(s) with hot water after each use, then pour isopropyl rubbing alcohol through them to sterilize. Allow to dry before using again.

Food Processor (full-size or small model). This can be used for mixing larger amounts of creams and lotions, or for making finely ground oatmeal, almond meal, and sunflower seed meal. Entire facial/body scrub recipes can be prepared in a food processor.

Note: If you don't currently own this piece of equipment, and decide to purchase one, make sure it is easy to clean. There are many models (mine included) that have sandwiched layers of plastic on various parts of the bowl and top that catch all sorts of seeds and food debris that *cannot* be removed, no matter how hard you try. Please look at several designs before you buy, and choose the one that is the easiest to clean.

Funnel (small). This comes in handy when pouring liquid recipes into narrow-necked storage bottles. Funnels can be made from aluminum foil in a snap. Because herbal liquids pass through funnels so quickly, there is no real risk of aluminum leaching as there is with aluminum pots.

Measuring Cups & Spoons. Self explanatory.

Mortar and Pestle (larger size — approximately 6" [15.24 cm] diameter). I use this tool to crush fennel seeds, to mash fresh herbs and flowers to a pulp to extract their fresh juices, and to make a mush of ripe papaya, pineapple chunks, or strawberry slices. A mortar and pestle is also handy for mixing essential oils with unscented powder mixtures when making herbal body powders.

Nut/seed grinder. I use this to grind oatmeal, almonds, and sunflower seeds into the precise texture I want. A small coffee grinder works equally well. Be sure to wipe out thoroughly after use.

Pans (1-, 2-, and 3-quart [946-ml, 1.9-l, and 2.8-l] enamel, glass, or stainless steel). Please *do not use* aluminum or copper pans. These metals can react with the herbs and acid liquids in your recipes and leach the aluminum or copper into the cosmetic you're making. Aluminum, in particular, is not good for your skin. It can also affect the beneficial qualities of the herbs and can discolor the end product.

Scale (tabletop or diet scale). When I first began making cosmetics, I used my scale constantly. Now, I can usually judge by "sight" the amount of an ingredient I'm measuring. However, I still rely on my scale when weighing out heavier herbs, such as roots, stems, seeds, and bark. If you can buy herbs by the ounce, a scale may be unnecessary.

Spatula (small and medium). These are perfect for scooping out creams and lotions from any type of container.

Spoons (wooden). You really need only two — one small and one medium-sized spoon. I use these for everything that needs stirring. If my whisk is dirty, I'll use a spoon for whipping my creams and lotions. They're indispensable.

Strainer (mesh). This is used to strain herbs and flowers from liquids in various recipes. Cheesecloth, panty hose, or coarsely woven burlap can substitute for a mesh strainer.

Whisk (small). I use this for whipping and blending almost all of my creams, lotions, and lip balms. It works best for blending small amounts versus the blender or food processor, which work better for larger recipes.

FOR STORING

Bottles (4 oz. to 16 oz.). I use either glass or plastic. Bottles are good for storing anything liquid, from astringents and toners to shampoos and mouthwashes. I recommend using brown, green, or blue glass if the cosmetic will be exposed to bright light for an extended period of time. Dark glass helps preserve the volatile oils in the herbs.

Low Tub or Jar (glass or plastic). All types of cosmetics can be stored in these containers. I keep all my creams, dentifrices, and lip balms in small containers with tight-fitting lids. Baby food jars make good containers, too.

Shaker Jar (glass or plastic). Use this for herbal body powders. The grocery store I frequent sells generic spices in 2½" (6 cm) diameter, 2.25 oz. (64 grams) capacity plastic shaker containers. After using the spice, I wash these thoroughly and save for my powders. I sometimes store dry facial and body scrub mixtures in them.

Spritzer. Good for astringents, toners, and insect repellents. Save and wash hairspray bottles for this purpose.

Squirt Bottle. Great for shampoos and conditioners, bath and massage oils, and astringents. Recycled dish detergent, shampoo, and castile soap bottles work great.

Tin. A tin is handy for storing any leftover dry herbs you may have on hand. They're relatively airtight and keep the bugs and light out. Also good for storing dry scrub, mask, powder, and bath mixtures.

RECYCLING STORAGE CONTAINERS:

If you plan to recycle previously used glass and plastic containers for storage purposes, please be sure to wash them thoroughly first. You can either run them through the dishwasher or allow them to soak in hot, soapy water for 10 minutes, scrub thoroughly, rinse, and allow to dry completely. Do not store your cosmetics in containers that previously held medicine, poisons, household cleansers (other than dishwashing liquid), spoiled foods, or fertilizer. Use your own good judgment about what containers are and are not safe to use.

Zip-Seal Freezer Bags. Perfect for storing scrubs or excess body powder if you've made a large quantity. Leftover dried herbs can be stored in these and kept in a dry, cool, dark place for several months.

FOR APPLYING

Tissues. Used primarily for blotting excess perspiration and oil from the face and for blotting or removing lipstick. Use only 100% cotton, unscented, white tissues. Dyes and deodorants may irritate delicate skin.

Cotton Balls/Cotton Squares. These can be soaked with oil to remove stubborn eye makeup, used to apply astringent or toner, or moistened with cleanser to cleanse the face and neck. I prefer to buy 100% cotton squares or cut my own from rolled cotton sometimes called "beautician's" cotton. Rolled cotton can be purchased from your local drug store or beauty supply store.

Complexion Brush. These brushes are usually about the size of your palm or may have a short handle with the bristles forming a circular pattern at the end. The bristles should be very soft and can be either synthetic or natural. Use a complexion brush much as you would a wash cloth, but stay away from the eye area.

Loofah Sponge. A loofah is actually the dried skeleton of a gourd. Available at most health food and drug stores, they're excellent for removing dried skin from the body but are too rough for facial use.

Pumice Stone or Powder. Volcanic rock or powder, pumice consists mainly of silicates. Rubbed on the knees, feet, elbows and hands, the rock is excellent for removing dry skin and callouses. Pumice powder is sometimes used in facial and body scrubs. Many commercial soaps designed to remove grease and oil stains from hands contain pumice powder.

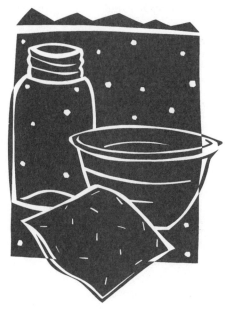

All-Natural
Cosmetic
Recipes

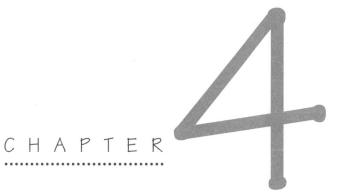

CHAPTER

In the sections that follow, you will find recipes for making natural personal care products for the face, body, hair, and more. The ingredients are quite easy to find and the recipes are relatively simple to make.

All herbs used in the following recipes are *dried* unless otherwise specified. If you have access to fresh herbs, then you may want to dry the herbs yourself (see page 9 for instructions). Recently dried herbs have a wonderful, just-picked aroma and will make your products all the more delightful.

A "recipe key," to the right of each ingredient list, gives a quick summary of the recipe as well as some added tips. Use it at a glance to tell whether that particular cosmetic is right for your skin or hair type.

MAKING MEAL BLENDS

Three of the main ingredients you will always want to have on hand are almond meal, ground oatmeal, and sunflower seed meal.

Almond Meal

To make a half-cup (118 ml) of *almond meal*, blend approximately 50 large, raw almonds in the blender or food processor until the consistency is like finely grated parmesan cheese.

Ground Oatmeal

To make one-half cup (118 ml) of *ground oatmeal*, blend one cup of old-fashioned oats in the blender or food processor until it feels like fine flour.

Sunflower Seed Meal

To make one-half cup (118 ml) of *sunflower seed meal*, grind ¾ cup (177 ml) of large seeds (hulled), until the consistency is also like parmesan cheese.

These measurements are only approximate because of size variations in the nuts, seeds, and oats.

HERBS AND INGREDIENTS THAT MAY CAUSE IRRITATION TO EYES AND SKIN

Almond, bitter, essential oil
Aloe Vera, skin of fresh leaf and gel
Benzoin, tincture of
Chamomile
Cinnamon, essential oil
Clove, essential oil
Cocoa Butter
Cornstarch
Glycerin
Lanolin
Lemon, essential oil
Lemongrass, essential oil
Lime, essential oil
Orange, essential oil
Synthetic essential oils
Tangerine, essential oil
Vinegar

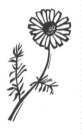

A FEW WORDS ABOUT SAFETY

Many of the recipes you make will look and smell edible because the majority of ingredients used will be edible. This does not mean that your skin or hair care products are safe to consume, though. Please, for safety's (and your taste-buds') sake, clearly label all your skin care products and keep out of the reach of children.

If you are allergy prone, it's best to test yourself for adverse reactions to the herbs called for in the recipe you're planning to use. To do this, try a patch test. Prepare a paste with 1 teaspoon (5 ml) of the herb in question and a small amount of boiling water. Apply the paste to cleaned skin on the inside of your elbow. Cover with an adhesive bandage and leave on for 24 hours. If it is an essential oil you are concerned about, dilute one drop with one tablespoon of water, saturate a cotton ball, and apply the same way as the paste. If a rash or redness appears, do not use this herb. Substitute with another that causes no reaction. (See the ingredient listing in chapter 2 for possible substitutes.)

If, while making your cosmetics, any of the solutions enter your eyes and an irritation develops, promptly flood your eyes with cool water repeatedly. If the irritation continues, see your physician as soon as possible.

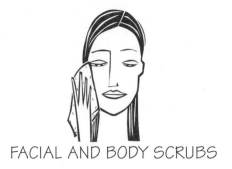

FACIAL AND BODY SCRUBS

A cosmetic scrub is used to remove dry, dead skin cells from the surface of the skin. It can be used on all skin types *except* those with severe acne, thread (spider) veins, or highly sensitive skin. A scrub may be too irritating for these conditions. These recipes should be used on facial and body areas only, unless otherwise specified.

Please note: When using any of these exfoliants, do not "scrub" your face and neck. Your body may be able to tolerate a bit more friction, but your delicate facial and neck skin cannot. Please allow the product to do the work for you and be very gentle.

For the face: Using a light touch with your fingers or a facial cloth, massage your face and neck in a circular, upward motion. Do this for approximately 1 minute. Rinse thoroughly. Avoid eye area at all times!

For the body: Scrubs may be applied to your body simply by using your hands or you may wish to use a body loofah, washcloth, or body brush. Use whatever feels best to you. I prefer to use the body scrubs in the shower, as they tend to be a bit messy.

GIFT IDEA

Facial and body scrubs make great gifts for men or women. Make up a cup or two of the scrub that best suits the recipient's skin type, put it in a regular plastic food storage bag, tie with a ribbon or twine, and place in a decorative tin, box, or gift bag with a nice note. Make sure you include complete instructions with your gift.

ALL-PURPOSE SCRUB

½ cup (118 ml) ground
  oatmeal
⅓ cup (79 ml) ground
  sunflower seeds
4 tablespoons (59 ml)
  almond meal
½ teaspoon (2.5 ml)
  ground peppermint,
  spearmint, or rosemary
  leaves
dash cinnamon powder
  (optional)
water, milk, or heavy cream

Good for: all skin types
Use: daily or as needed
Follow with: moisturizer
Prep time: approximately 10 minutes
Mix with: blender, food processor
Store in: zip-seal bag, low tub/jar, or tin
Yields: 4 to 24 treatments, depending on use
Special: Leaves skin very smooth.

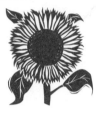

Mix dry ingredients together thoroughly. Use approximately 2 teaspoons (10 ml) of scrub mixture for the face, more for the body, and enough water (for oily skin), milk (for normal skin), or heavy cream (for dry skin), to form a spreadable paste. Allow to thicken for 1 minute. Massage onto face and throat or body area. Rinse.

GENTLE FACIAL EXFOLIANT

2 tablespoons (30 ml)
  powdered milk
½ cup (118 ml) ground
  oatmeal
1 teaspoon (5 ml) cornmeal
water

Good for: all skin types, especially dry and
sensitive
Use: daily or as needed
Follow with: moisturizer
Prep time: approximately 5 minutes
Mix with: small bowl and spoon
Store in: zip-seal bag, low tub/jar, or tin
Yields: approximately 10 treatments
Special: Leaves skin silky soft.

Mix dry ingredients thoroughly. Combine 1 tablespoon (15 ml) of scrub mixture with enough water to form a spreadable paste. Allow to thicken for 1 minute. Massage onto face and throat. Rinse.

SCRUB FOR OILY SKIN

½ cup (118 ml) ground
    oatmeal
½ cup (118 ml) almond
    meal
1 tablespoon (15 ml) sea
    salt
1 teaspoon (5 ml) ground
    peppermint leaves
1 teaspoon (5 ml) ground
    rosemary leaves
astringent of choice (see
    recipes)

Good for: normal and oily skin
Use: three times per week
Follow with: astringent, then moisturizer
Prep time: approximately 10 minutes
Mix with: blender or food processor
Store in: zip-seal bag, low tub/jar, or tin
Yields: approximately 16 treatments
Special: Great for oily areas on shoulders, chest, and back.

Thoroughly mix all dry ingredients. Mix 1 tablespoon (15 ml) of scrub with enough astringent to form a paste. Allow to thicken. Massage *gently* onto face and throat. Rinse.

BODY SCRUB

¼ cup (59 ml) sea salt
¼ cup (59 ml) warmed
    coconut or olive oil

Good for: all skin types
Use: as desired
Follow with: moisturizer, if desired
Prep time: approximately 5 minutes
Mix with: small bowl and spoon
Store in: Make recipe only as needed. Do not store.
Yields: 1 treatment
Special: Leaves calloused areas especially soft.

Stir both ingredients together. Massage onto body with hands or mitt using a light, but firm, pressure. Continue massaging, *not rubbing,* until a rosy glow appears. Rinse with warm water, towel dry.

CREAMY SCRUB CLEANSER

2 tablespoons (30 ml) heavy cream (or 1 tbsp. [15 ml] cream and 1 tbsp. [15 ml] peach pureé)

1 tablespoon (15 ml) ground oatmeal

1 teaspoon (5 ml) sunflower seed meal

½ teaspoon (2.5 ml) chamomile flowers

Good for: normal and dry skin
Use: daily or as desired
Follow with: moisturizer
Prep time: 5 to 10 minutes
Mix with: mortar and pestle or small bowl and fork
Store in: Dry mix: zip-seal bag, low tub/jar, or tin
Yields: 1 treatment
Special: May use as mask — allow to dry 15 to 20 minutes. Rinse. Very soothing.

Mix ingredients together to form a very creamy paste. Massage onto face and throat. Allow mixture to remain on your face for approximately 5 minutes. Rinse. Used frequently, your skin should acquire a "peaches and cream" glow!

ALMOND MEAL CLEANSER

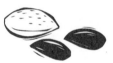

½ cup (118 ml) almond meal

water, milk, or heavy cream

Good for: all skin types
Use: daily or as desired
Follow with: moisturizer
Prep time: approximately 5 minutes
Mix with: small bowl and spoon
Store in: Dry mix: zip-seal bag, low tub/jar, or tin
Yields: approximately 12 treatments

Mix 2 teaspoons (10 ml) of almond meal with enough liquid to form a paste. Spread onto moistened face and throat and gently massage for 1 minute. Rinse with warm water.

OATMEAL SMOOTHER

½ cup (118 ml) ground
  oatmeal
½ cup (118 ml) powdered
  milk
water

Good for: all skin types, especially dry, deli-
cate, sensitive skin
Use: daily or as desired
Follow with: moisturizer
Prep time: approximately 5 minutes
Mix with: small bowl and spoon
Store in: Dry mix: zip-seal bag, low tub/jar,
or tin
Yields: approximately 24 treatments
Special: Leaves skin very smooth and soft.

Mix 2 teaspoons (10 ml) of scrub mixture with 2 teaspoons (10 ml) water. Stir until a smooth paste forms. Massage onto face and throat. Rinse.

BALANCING SCRUB

1 tablespoon (15 ml)
  papaya pulp or plain
  yogurt
2 teaspoons (10 ml)
  ground oatmeal
1 teaspoon (5 ml) sea salt

Good for: oily and normal-to-dry skin
Use: two times per week
Follow with: moisturizer
Prep time: approximately 5 minutes
Mix with: small bowl and fork
Store in: Make recipe only as needed. Do not
store.
Yields: 1 treatment
Special: Good for blotchy or unevenly colored
skin.

Combine ingredients and massage mixture onto face and throat until a rosy glow appears. Leave on for 5 minutes. Rinse with cool water. Use this scrub every week until your skin begins to become more uniformly colored and has attained a smooth appearance.

SENSATIONAL SUNFLOWER FRICTION

1 tablespoon (15 ml)
   sunflower seed meal
1 tablespoon (15 ml)
   applesauce

Good for: normal and dry skin
Use: three times per week
Follow with: moisturizer
Prep time: approximately 5 minutes
Mix with: small bowl and spoon
Store in: Do not store. Mix only as needed.
Yields: 1 treatment
Special: Very moisturizing.

Combine ingredients to form a paste. Massage onto face and throat. Allow to remain for 10 minutes so that the oils of the sunflower seeds may be released and absorbed into your thirsty skin. Rinse with warm water.

PINEAPPLE/SUNFLOWER SCRUB

1 tablespoon (15 ml) sun-
   flower seed meal
1 tablespoon (15 ml) fresh
   pineapple or lemon juice
   (diluted 50% with
   water)

Good for: oily and normal-to-dry skin
Use: two times per week
Follow with: moisturizer
Prep time: 5 to 10 minutes
Mix with: small bowl and spoon
Store in: Do not store. Mix only as needed.
Yields: 1 treatment
Special: Excellent for a fading tan. Evens skin tone.

Mix ingredients thoroughly and massage onto face and throat. Include the chest area if skin tone is uneven there. Allow to dry for 10 minutes. Rinse with cool water. This scrub tends to bleach the skin slightly. Use every week until your skin takes on a smooth, even appearance.

CORNMEAL AND HONEY SCRUB

1½ teaspoons (7.5 ml) cornmeal
½ teaspoon (2.5 ml) water
1 teaspoon (5 ml) honey

Good for: all skin types, except sensitive
Use: three times per week
Follow with: moisturizer
Prep time: approximately 5 minutes
Mix with: small bowl and spoon
Store in: Do not store. Mix only as needed.
Yields: 1 treatment

Combine ingredients thoroughly and allow to thicken for 1 minute. Massage onto face and throat and leave on for 15 minutes. Rinse with warm water.

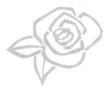

BREWER'S YEAST AND OATMEAL SCRUB

¼ cup (59 ml) brewer's
  yeast (not baking
  yeast)
¼ cup (59 ml) ground
  oatmeal
water

Good for: oily and normal-to-dry skin

Use: two times per week

Follow with: moisturizer

Prep time: approximately 5 minutes

Mix with: small bowl and spoon

Store in: Dry mix: zip-seal bag, low tub/jar, or tin

Yields: approximately 8 treatments

Special: Revs up the circulation — great for a pale complexion!

Mix dry ingredients completely. Using 1 tablespoon (15 ml) scrub and approximately 1 tablespoon (15 ml) water, form a spreadable paste. Allow to thicken for 1 minute. Massage onto face and throat and allow to dry for 15 minutes. Rinse with cool water.

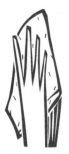

CLEANSING CREAMS AND LOTIONS

*C*leansing creams and lotions are used to remove makeup and everyday dirt and grime that collects in your facial pores. Unlike using soap to cleanse your face, which has a tendency to dry the skin's surface, these products are very gentle and nourishing and do a thorough job of cleansing.

Application tip: First, moisten your face and throat with a warm, moist washcloth or several splashes of warm water. Next, apply a small amount of cleanser (about a teaspoon or two [5 to 10 ml] will do) using the pads of your fingers, with upward, circular strokes. Continue applying cleanser until your entire facial area is covered. Now, gently remove cleanser with a moistened washcloth, then splash your face several times with clean, warm water. Pat dry. You are now ready to apply the appropriate toner or astringent for your skin type.

Important "cooking" instructions: Many of the following recipes require the heating of various oils, waxes, and other ingredients so that they may be properly blended. When "cooking" your cleansing creams and lotions, please use the "low" setting on your stove to warm or melt your ingredients or use a double boiler. *Never* let the herbal liquid or wax/oil mixture get hot. *Warm* them just enough for the waxes to melt and the borax to dissolve in the herbal liquid. Both the wax/oil and the herbal liquid/borax mixtures should be approximately the same temperature when

GIFT IDEA

Freshly made cleansing creams, along with the appropriate toner and moisturizer make a nice complete skin care gift. Bottle products in glass containers, such as French jelly jars, or small jars with cork tops. Label each cosmetic with a decorative sticker. Line a small basket with a brightly colored face cloth, sprinkle a few tablespoons of lavender, or rose petals along the bottom, and place your cosmetics inside. Tie a ribbon around the basket. Print complete instructions for each cosmetic on nice stationery and include it in an envelope or in scroll form with a ribbon.

See Astringents and Toners for suggestion on how to bottle herbal tonics.

blending together. If one mixture is much warmer than the other, the end product may separate or feel lumpy or grainy.

Here's another hint: to make a product thicker or firmer, add more beeswax or cocoa butter. To soften, add more oil or herbal liquid and a pinch of borax.

ALOE AND CALENDULA CLEANSING LOTION

2 tablespoons (30 ml) aloe
vera gel
1 tablespoon (15 ml) strong
calendula or chamomile
tea
4 tablespoons (59 ml)
avocado, sweet almond,
castor, or grapeseed oil
1 tablespoon (15 ml)
beeswax
¼ teaspoon (1.25 ml)
borax
fifty thousand international units vitamin A (cap-
sules)
5 drops essential oil of
carrot seed, sandal-
wood, marjoram, or
geranium

Good for: normal and dry skin
Use: daily
Follow with: astringent or toner
Prep time: approximately 45 minutes
Mix with: whisk
Store in: low tub or jar
Yields: approximately 12 treatments
Special: Soothing and healing.

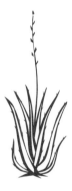

Melt together oil and beeswax in a small pan or double boiler. Warm the tea and aloe vera gel in another pan and stir in borax until borax is dissolved. Remove both pans from heat and slowly pour the herbal mixture into the wax/oil pan, beating steadily with your whisk until cool, thick, and smooth. Pierce the vitamin A capsules and squeeze contents into lotion. Add essential oil. Blend completely one more time before storing. Use approximately 2 teaspoons (10 ml) per application. Does not require refrigeration if used up within 30 days, or unless weather is very hot.

BASIC COLD CREAM

1 ounce (30 ml) virgin olive, jojoba, sweet almond, apricot kernel, or avocado oil

4 ounces (120 ml) pure vegetable shortening (no lard, please!)

5 drops tincture of benzoin

5 drops of your favorite essential oil

Good for: normal and dry skin
Use: daily
Follow with: astringent/toner
Prep time: approximately 30 minutes
Mix with: whisk
Store in: low tub or jar
Yields: approximately 15 treatments
Special: Makes a great overnight treatment for hands or feet. Make sure you wear gloves or socks to bed!

Warm the oil and shortening in a small pan or double boiler until completely melted together. Remove from heat and stir in the tincture of benzoin and essential oil. Allow to cool a bit, then begin whisking until cool, thick, and creamy. Store. Use approximately 2 teaspoons (10 ml) per application. Product performs best if used within 30 days; otherwise, refrigerate.

HERBAL SOAPY SKIN WASH

16-ounce (480 ml) bottle plain castile liquid soap

5 drops essential oil of tea tree

5 drops essential oil of peppermint

3 drops essential oil of lemon balm (also called melissa)

5 drops essential oil of chamomile, German, or essential oil of sandalwood

1 teaspoon (5 ml) sweet almond, jojoba, or grapeseed oil

Good for: normal and oily skin
Use: daily
Follow with: astringent or toner
Prep time: approximately 10 minutes
Mix with: shake before use
Store in: castile soap bottle
Yields: approximately 32 treatments
Special: This makes an especially invigorating body wash, too!

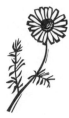

Add the drops of essential oils and teaspoon of oil to the bottle of castile soap. Shake vigorously. Use 1 tablespoon (15 ml) per application.

CLEANSING AND REJUVENATING OIL

2 tablespoons (30 ml)
  each: melted coconut,
  apricot kernel, avocado
  or sunflower, grapeseed,
  jojoba, sweet almond,
  and virgin olive oils
five thousand international
  units vitamin E oil
5 drops essential oil of
  carrot seed, sandal-
  wood, lavender, or rosemary

Good for: all skin types
Use: daily
Follow with: astringent or toner
Prep time: 10 to 15 minutes
Mix with: spoon and small bowl
Store in: bottle
Yields: approximately 42 treatments
Special: Effectively removes eye makeup, even
stubborn waterproof types!

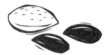

Combine all ingredients and store. Requires no refrigeration if used up within 30 days. Shake well before each use of approximately 1 teaspoon (5 ml) per application.

This special oil blend nourishes dry, parched skin and maintains the glow of normal, healthy skin. Oily skins can benefit from the nourishment of these healing oils, too, but make sure to apply the appropriate astringent following cleansing to remove any oil residue.

CLASSIC ROSEWATER AND GLYCERIN CLEANSER

½ cup (118 ml) rosewater
½ cup (118 ml) glycerin

Good for: normal and dry skin
Use: daily
Follow with: astringent and toner
Prep time: approximately 15 minutes
Mix with: shake before each use
Store in: bottle
Yields: 16 treatments
Special: Very gentle and soothing.

Combine ingredients and heat to just boiling. *Do not allow to boil.* Store. Apply this liquid cleanser with a washcloth or cotton pads. Use 1 tablespoon (15 ml) per application. Refrigeration not required.

LEMON CLEANSER

2 tablespoons (30 ml)
strained lemon juice

¼ cup (59 ml) plus 1 tablespoon (15 ml) grapeseed
or apricot kernel oil

1 tablespoon (15 ml)
beeswax

¼ teaspoon (1.25 ml)
borax

6 drops essential oil of
lemon or tangerine

Good for: normal or oily skin

Use: daily

Follow with: astringent or toner

Prep time: approximately 45 minutes

Mix with: whisk

Store in: low tub or jar

Yields: approximately 9 treatments

In a small pan or double boiler, melt the oil and wax. Warm the lemon juice in another small pan and stir in borax until dissolved. Remove both pans from heat and slowly combine mixtures while beating steadily with your whisk until cool and creamy. Add essential oil and stir thoroughly. Store in refrigerator if not used up within 2 weeks or if house is very warm. Use 2 teaspoons (10 ml) per application.

STRAWBERRY CLEANSER

4 very ripe medium-sized
strawberries, sliced

2 drops essential oil of
yarrow or peppermint

Good for: normal or oily skin

Use: daily — when strawberries are in season

Follow with: astringent or toner

Prep time: 5 to 10 minutes

Mix with: mortar and pestle, spoon

Store in: Do not store. Mix only as needed.

Yields: 1 treatment

Special: The strawberry juice can also serve as a tooth cleanser and whitener. Very refreshing!

Mash the strawberries and press through mesh strainer or squeeze through cheesecloth or panty hose. Catch juice in a small condiment bowl. Add essential oil and stir to blend. Apply to face and neck with a saturated cotton square and massage with finger tips for about 1 minute. Avoid eye area. Rinse with cool water.

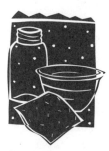

ASTRINGENTS AND TONERS

Astringents and toners, by definition, are agents used to remove the last traces of cleanser residue and also to remove excess perspiration and oil.

Astringents tend to be the stronger of the two and are usually used for normal-to-oily and oily skin types. Many commercial astringents contain alcohol and/or acetone (nail polish remover), which are very drying and damaging to the skin's surface. Herbal astringents tend to be gentler and are preferable to a chemical-based product.

Toners, on the other hand, perform the same function as an astringent but are designed for the normal-to-dry and dry skin. Thus, toners are milder by design and do not remove as much surface oil.

Storage tip: All of the following astringent and toner recipes should be stored in the refrigerator to preserve freshness unless otherwise indicated. Chemical preservatives have not been used in these recipes to extend the shelf life of the product. Please store your products in tightly sealed and labeled bottles or spritzers.

Application tip: Astringents and toners should be applied to the face and neck with a 100% cotton ball or pad in upward strokes. Always follow the use of these products with an appropriate moisturizer for your skin type.

GIFT IDEA

Who wouldn't appreciate receiving a freshly made herbal facial tonic packaged in a colored glass or decorative vinegar bottle topped with a cork? What a creative and useful gift! To make it even nicer, add a fresh sprig or peel of the herb called for in the recipe to the bottle. This just adds to the aesthetic appeal. Add a decorative label with instructions for use and make sure to note if it needs to be refrigerated.

LEMON REFRESHER

Juice of half a lemon
½ cup (118 ml) witch hazel
(commercially prepared
is fine)

Good for: oily skin
Use: daily
Follow with: moisturizer
Prep time: approximately 5 minutes
Mix with: cup or bowl and spoon
Store in: bottle or spritzer
Yields: approximately 24 treatments
Special: Very refreshing.

Mix ingredients, store, and shake well before each use. Use approximately 1 teaspoon (5 ml) per application.

PARSLEY AND PEPPERMINT ASTRINGENT

¼ cup (59 ml) fresh
chopped parsley
¼ cup (59 ml) fresh pep-
permint leaves or 2
tablespoons (30 ml)
dried
1 cup (237 ml) distilled
water
10 drops tincture of ben-
zoin

Good for: normal and oily skin
Use: daily
Follow with: moisturizer
Prep time: approximately 35 minutes
Mix with: shake before use
Store in: bottle or spritzer
Yields: approximately 48 treatments

Bring water to boil and remove from heat. Add herbs and allow to steep for 30 minutes. Keep the lid on the pot while steeping. Add tincture of benzoin. Strain and store. Each week make a new solution. Use approximately 1 teaspoon (5 ml) per application.

pH RESTORER

▼▼▼▼▼

2 cups (473 ml) distilled
  water
¼ cup (59 ml) apple cider
  vinegar
10 drops favorite essential
  oil — try lavender,
  lemon, or rose

Good for: all skin types
Use: daily
Follow with: moisturizer
Prep time: approximately 5 to 10 minutes
Mix with: shake before use
Store in: bottle or spritzer
Yields: approximately 32 treatments
Special: Softens skin.

Combine ingredients and store. Use approximately 1 tablespoon (15 ml) per application. Splash it on if you wish. The vinegar will help combat the alkaline residue that soap or cleansers can leave behind. When your skin maintains the correct pH balance (5.5), it has a much better chance of fighting off infections. Requires no refrigeration.

OLD-FASHIONED LAVENDER TONER

▼▼▼▼▼

1 tablespoon (15 ml) lavender flowers
1 cup (237 ml) witch hazel
6 drops essential oil of
  lavender

Good for: normal and dry skin
Use: daily
Follow with: moisturizer
Prep time: 2 weeks
Mix with: shake jar occasionally during
2-week period
Store in: bottle or spritzer
Yields: approximately 48 treatments
Special: Smells sweet and floral.

Combine ingredients in a tightly lidded jar and store in a dark, cool place. Allow lavender to steep for 2 weeks. Shake jar vigorously every other day or so. Strain and bottle. Use approximately 1 teaspoon (5 ml) per application and shake well before each use. Requires no refrigeration.

FENNEL SOOTHER

1 tablespoon (15 ml) crushed fennel seeds

¼ cup (59 ml) apple cider vinegar

2 cups (473 ml) distilled water

2 teaspoons (10 ml) glycerin

Good for: all skin types, especially rashy and irritated

Use: daily

Follow with: moisturizer

Prep time: 50 to 55 minutes

Mix with: mortar and pestle to crush seeds

Store in: bottle or spritzer

Yields: approximately 32 treatments

Special: Softens skin and hair, if used as a rinse; restores pH.

Boil water. Remove from heat and add crushed fennel seeds. Allow to steep for 45 minutes. Strain, add glycerin and vinegar, and store. Shake well before each use. Use 1 tablespoon (15 ml) per application; splash on if desired. Does not require refrigeration if product is used up within 30 days.

ACNE ASTRINGENT

1 tablespoon (15 ml) yarrow

1 tablespoon (15 ml) calendula or chamomile

2 cups (473 ml) distilled water

15 drops tincture of benzoin

6 drops essential oil of peppermint

Good for: oily skin

Use: daily

Follow with: moisturizer

Prep time: approximately 35 minutes

Mix with: shake before use

Store in: bottle or spritzer

Yields: approximately 96 treatments

Special: Healing and soothing.

Bring water to a boil. Remove from heat and add herbs. Cover and steep for 30 minutes. Strain. Add tincture of benzoin and peppermint oil. Store. Use 1 teaspoon (5 ml) per application. Refrigerate.

ALOE VERA TONER

Pure aloe vera gel

Good for: normal and oily skin (those with sensitive skin, see *Note* below)
Use: daily
Follow with: moisturizer
Prep time: none
Mix with: n/a
Store in: n/a
Special: Great overall toner. Also relieves burns, sunburn, itch from insect bites.

Simply soak a cotton pad with the gel and use to freshen skin and remove excess oil. Follow directions on label regarding storage. If you use a leaf from your aloe plant, cut off the amount you are going to use and *put the remainder of the leaf in a plastic bag and store* in the refrigerator. Leaf will keep for about 3 days.

Note: Aloe juice may irritate sensitive skin. You can lessen the irritating effects by diluting the gel 50/50 with distilled or spring water. Store in small jar and shake vigorously before application. Keep refrigerated.

TANGERINE TONER

½ cup (118 ml) witch hazel
6 drops essential oil of
tangerine

Good for: normal and oily skin
Use: daily
Follow with: moisturizer
Prep time: 5 minutes
Mix with: shake before use
Store in: bottle or spritzer
Yields: approximately 24 treatments

Combine ingredients and shake vigorously. Store. Use 1 teaspoon (5 ml) per application. Requires no refrigeration.

HERBAL ASTRINGENT

1 cup (237 ml) distilled
   water
½ cup (118 ml) pure vodka
1 teaspoon (5 ml) each:
   sage, yarrow,
   chamomile, rosemary,
   lemon balm, peppermint,
   spearmint, and straw-
   berry leaves
¼ cup (59 ml) witch hazel

Good for: oily and normal skin
Use: daily
Follow with: moisturizer
Prep time: 2 weeks
Mix with: shake jar occasionally during 2-week period
Store in: bottle or spritzer
Yields: approximately 84 treatments
Special: Great following exercise! Thoroughly removes all oil and perspiration.

Mix ingredients thoroughly and store for 2 weeks in a tightly sealed jar. Keep in a cool, dark place. Strain. Refrigeration is not required, though a cool product is nice on a hot summer day! Use 1 teaspoon (5 ml) per application.

MINTY ASTRINGENT

1 tablespoon (15 ml) fresh
   peppermint, spearmint,
   or lemon balm (if dried,
   use 1½ teaspoons (7.5
   ml) of herb
1 cup (237 ml) witch hazel

Good for: normal and oily skin
Use: daily
Follow with: moisturizer
Prep time: 1 week
Mix with: shake jar occasionally during the week
Store in: bottle or spritzer
Yields: approximately 48 treatments
Special: Has a nice fragrance. Could be used by men as an aftershave.

Combine the ingredients in a jar with a tight-fitting lid. Allow herb to steep for 1 week. Strain. Use 1 teaspoon (5 ml) per application. Refrigeration not required.

ORANGE FLOWER TONER

1 tablespoon (15 ml) orange flowers

1 teaspoon (5 ml) rose petals

2 tablespoons (30 ml) glycerin

1 cup (237 ml) distilled water

Good for: normal and dry skin
Use: daily
Follow with: moisturizer if necessary
Prep time: 50 to 55 minutes
Mix with: spoon or whisk, small bowl
Store in: bottle or spritzer
Yields: approximately 54 treatments
Special: Very gentle and soothing.

Bring water to a boil and remove from heat. Add herbs and steep for 45 minutes in a covered pot. Strain. Slowly add glycerin, stirring constantly. Store. Use 1 teaspoon (5 ml) per application. Shake vigorously before each use.

ELDER FLOWER TONER

1 tablespoon (15 ml) elder flowers

1 cup (237 ml) distilled water

1 tablespoon (15 ml) glycerin

5 drops essential oil of sandalwood or lavender (optional)

Good for: normal and dry skin
Use: daily
Follow with: moisturizer if necessary
Prep time: 50 to 55 minutes
Mix with: spoon or whisk, small bowl
Store in: bottle or spritzer
Yields: approximately 50 treatments
Special: Super for extra dry skin, especially if oil of sandalwood is used.

Bring water to a boil and remove from heat. Add herb and steep for 45 minutes in a covered pot. Strain. Slowly add glycerin and essential oil, stirring constantly. Store. Use 1 teaspoon (5 ml) per application. Shake vigorously before each use.

SPICY AFTERSHAVE

2 cups (473 ml) witch
    hazel
1 sprig fresh rosemary
1 sprig fresh mint of choice
1 cinnamon stick
5 to 10 whole cloves
2 strips fresh orange peel
    cut into spirals
2 strips fresh lemon peel
    cut into spirals
15 drops tincture of
    benzoin

Good for: all skin types, except very dry
Use: daily or as desired
Follow with: moisturizer
Prep time: 2 weeks
Mix with: shake bottle gently every 2 days
Store in: decorative bottle
Yields: approximately 12 splashes
Special: When strained, can be used as a
scented hair rinse for normal or oily dark hair.

Place all of the ingredients and tincture of benzoin in a decorative bottle with the witch hazel. Cap tightly and store for 2 weeks. Leave the herbs and other ingredients in the bottle. Smells delightful! Use approximately 2½ tablespoons (37.5 ml) per application, or more if you like.

Note: Use organically grown fruit — if available — to avoid pesticide residue. Be sure to wash fruit thoroughly.

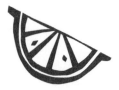

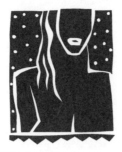

MOISTURIZING CREAMS AND LOTIONS

Moisturizers can be your skin's best friend! By applying a moisturizer to your skin, you are, in effect, putting a barrier between your skin and a world full of pollutants, drying air-conditioning and heat in your home or office, and the aging effects of the sun. Always use a moisturizer designed for your skin type, otherwise your skin may look oily from over-moisturizing or be thirsty from under-moisturizing.

Application tip: Moisturizers should always be applied following the use of your toner or astringent and immediately following a facial treatment, such as a scrub, steam, or mask. Apply your moisturizer onto a freshly cleansed face that is still slightly damp from the toner, astringent, or rinse water. Using upward, circular motions, apply your moisturizer the same way as you would your cleanser. Wait one minute to allow your skin to "drink" the moisture, then proceed with your makeup or sunscreen. The moisturizer "seals in" the moisture already present on your skin and thus prevents your delicate facial tissue from dehydrating. By all means, don't forget to moisturize your neck and chest. Many women neglect these areas, which can actually reveal the aging effects of sun exposure and general neglect sooner than your face. Moisturizing is the last step in your skin care process.

Important "cooking" instructions: Please read this section detailed under *Cleansing Creams and Lotions* before you proceed with the following recipes.

COCOA BUTTER LOTION FOR FACE AND BODY

1 tablespoon (15 ml) cocoa
  butter
1 tablespoon (15 ml) anhydrous lanolin
⅔ cup (158 ml) grapeseed,
  sweet almond, apricot
  kernel, or jojoba oil
3 tablespoons (44 ml)
  distilled water
½ teaspoon (2.5 ml) borax
6 drops essential oil of
  sandalwood, fennel, or
  geranium

Good for: normal and dry skin
Use: daily
Prep time: approximately 45 minutes
Mix with: whisk
Store in: low tub or jar
Yields: approximately 25 treatments, depend-
ing on use

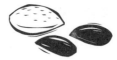

Melt together the cocoa butter, anhydrous lanolin, and oil in a small pan or double boiler. Heat the water in a separate pan and stir in borax until dissolved. Remove both from heat and slowly combine the mixtures, stirring with your whisk. Blend until cool and creamy. Add essential oil and blend again. Store. Use 2 or more teaspoons (10 ml) per application. Refrigeration not required if used up within 30 days.

LIGHT MOISTURIZER

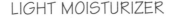

½ cup (118 ml) distilled
  water
3 teaspoons (15 ml)
  glycerin
5 drops essential oil of
  lemon

Good for: normal and oily skin
Use: daily
Prep time: approximately 5 minutes
Mix with: shake before use
Store in: bottle or spritzer
Yields: approximately 24 treatments

Pour ingredients into storage bottle and shake vigorously. Product can be applied using a cotton ball or by spraying the skin lightly and allowing to dry. Great to use anytime your skin needs refreshing or is feeling dehydrated. Use 1 teaspoon (5 ml) per application. Refrigeration not required.

PROTECTION CREAM

¼ cup (59 ml) pre-warmed
   coconut oil
½ cup (118 ml) sweet
   almond, extra-virgin
   olive, jojoba, or grapeseed oil
½ tablespoon (7.5 ml)
   cocoa butter

Good for: normal, dry, and severely chapped
skin
Use: as desired
Prep time: approximately 45 minutes
Mix with: whisk
Store in: low tub or jar
Yields: approximately 12 treatments
Special: Can be used as an intensive overnight
hand and foot cream.

Combine all ingredients in a small pan or double boiler and heat just until the
cocoa butter melts. Remove from heat. Allow mixture to cool slightly, then beat
vigorously, cool a bit more, then beat again until creamy.

I use this cream mainly on my body, especially on areas that need extra
attention. In the winter, I take a warm bath, pat dry, slather this cream on generously everywhere, then put on my long flannel gown and socks and go to bed.
My husband doesn't find this outfit attractive, by any means, but he does like
the way my skin feels the next morning. Use 1 tablespoon (15 ml), more or less,
per application. No need to refrigerate if used up within 30 days.

Note: Cream may harden in cold weather. To soften, place container in a
shallow pan of hot water for about 10 minutes.

ALOE AND CALENDULA CLEANSING LOTION
(see recipe under Cleansing Creams and Lotions, page 43)

This is one of my favorite all-purpose herbal lotions. I use it as a cleanser *and*
a moisturizer. It serves as a lightweight but very effective moisturizer for the
whole body. It is ideal for normal and dry skin, and is absorbed quickly without
leaving an oily residue. This lotion is perfect to take traveling when you can
only take a minimum of cosmetics.

BABY'S BOTTOM CREAM

2 teaspoons (10 ml) non-
petroleum jelly

2 teaspoons (10 ml) cocoa
butter

2 tablespoons (30 ml)
grapeseed, jojoba, or
castor oil

2 drops essential oil of
orange blossom, apple
blossom, carrot seed, or
lemon balm (melissa)

Good for: all skin types, especially normal
and dry

Use: as desired

Prep time: approximately 30 minutes

Mix with: whisk

Store in: low tub or jar

Yields: approximately 8 treatments

Special: Makes a great "ski cream"! Really pro-
tects against the dry, frigid air. Also makes a
good diaper rash prevention cream.

Heat all ingredients (except essential oil) in a small pan just until the cocoa butter is melted. Remove from heat and allow to cool a bit, then stir occasionally until cool and thick. Add essential oil, then beat again. Store. This cream will not turn white but will be relatively thick and clear. Use 1 teaspoon (5 ml) per application. Refrigeration not required.

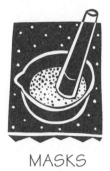

MASKS

The use of masks dates back to ancient civilizations that believed particular types of mud and clay, when applied to the body, had healing properties. Also, many tribes of people used clay which was tinted various colors. These specially prepared clays were painted onto the faces and bodies of tribe members to signify a particular event, such as a celebration or a war, was about to take place. Today, though, masks are used mainly to deep-clean, tone, or soften the skin, depending on the ingredients they contain.

Masks can be made from a myriad of natural ingredients, such as fuller's earth, French clay, or brewer's yeast, which absorb excess oil and dead cells from the skin's surface and stimulate a sluggish complexion. Masks can also be made from such succulent ingredients as fresh, ripe peaches and cream which moisturize a dry complexion and leave your skin with a wonderful "peaches and cream" glow. Try to set aside some personal time each week to devote to your skin. Relax and enjoy one of the following recipes. Your mind will appreciate the quiet time, and your skin will reward you with a renewed complexion!

Application tip: Masks should always be applied to freshly cleansed, damp skin. Begin at the neck and apply in an upward action. Remember to avoid applying the mask to the delicate eye area, as irritation may develop. Allow the mask to remain on your skin at least 20 minutes or longer, unless otherwise specified. Remove with a warm, wet washcloth, and apply moisturizer if necessary.

GIFT IDEA

There are several mask recipes that can be packaged and given as gifts. These include masks which are based on dry ingredients, such as clay, ground oatmeal, sunflower seed meal, wheat germ, brewer's yeast, and almond meal. Prepare a few of the base ingredients and measure approximately ½ cup (118 ml) of each and put into individual plastic bags, tightly sealed. Attach instructions for the mask to each bag with a ribbon. Place three or four bags inside a decorative tin or small wooden box.

BASIC CLAY MASK

½ cup (118 ml) French clay
   or fuller's earth
Cream — dry skin
Milk — normal skin
Water — oily skin

Good for: all skin types
Use: one to two times per week, or as desired
Follow with: moisturizer
Prep time: approximately 5 minutes
Mix with: small bowl and spoon
Store in: dry ingredient only — low tub/jar,
zip-seal bag, or tin
Yields: approximately 8 treatments

Combine 1 tablespoon (15 ml) of clay with enough of the appropriate liquid (determined by your skin type) to form a smooth, spreadable paste. Spread onto face and neck and allow to dry thoroughly. Rinse.

This mask can serve as an excellent overnight pimple treatment. Simply take a cotton swab and apply a dab on each pimple and leave on while you sleep. In the morning, rinse the remaining bits of mask with warm water. The clay absorbs the excess oil during the night and aids in the healing of the pimples.

EGG WHITE FIRMING MASK

White of 1 fresh egg
1 teaspoon (5 ml) corn-
   starch

Good for: normal and oily skin, especially
skin with large pores
Use: one time per week, or as desired
Follow with: moisturizer
Prep time: 5 to 10 minutes
Mix with: small bowl and whisk
Store in: Do not store. Mix as needed.
Yields: 1 treatment
Special: Minimizes the appearance of large
pores. Excellent skin tightener.

Combine the ingredients and beat until stiff peaks form. Smooth onto a clean face and allow to dry. Rinse. If you have a slant board, lie on this while your mask is drying. You'll swear you've had a mini face-lift when you're finished!

YOGURT ASTRINGENT/BLEACHING MASK

2 teaspoons (10 ml) plain
yogurt

Good for: normal, oily, and blotchy skin
Use: one to two times per week, or as desired
Follow with: moisturizer
Prep time: approximately 1 minute
Mix with: small bowl and spoon
Store in: keep yogurt refrigerated
Yields: 1 treatment
Special: Great for a fading tan, slightly bleaches and evens skin tone with repeated use.

Apply the yogurt to face and neck. Allow to dry, preferably while lying down. Rinse.

BREWER'S YEAST MASK

1 tablespoon (15 ml) brewer's yeast
1 tablespoon (15 ml) milk or
water

Good for: normal and oily skin
Use: one to two times per week
Follow with: moisturizer
Prep time: approximately 5 minutes
Mix with: small bowl and spoon
Store in: Do not store. Mix only as needed.
Yields: 1 treatment
Special: Brings a very rosy glow to the skin. Helps chase away that winter "pasty pale" look.

Combine ingredients to form a smooth paste. You may need more or less liquid than called for, depending on the brand of yeast used. Spread onto face in a thin layer, allow to dry, rinse. This mask may tingle as it dries. This is normal. If it starts to sting, rinse it off immediately and apply a good moisturizer.

PAPAYA "NO-MORE-PORES" DOUBLE MASK TREATMENT

¼ cup (59 ml) freshly
  mashed papaya
1 teaspoon (5 ml) fresh
  pineapple juice
  (optional)

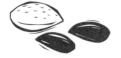

Good for: all skin types, except sensitive and sunburned
Use: one time per week
Follow with: moisturizer
Prep time: 5 to 10 minutes
Mix with: mortar and pestle, or small bowl and fork
Store in: Do not store. Mix as needed.
Yields: 1 treatment
Special: Mask is slightly bleaching and leaves a wonderful glow upon the skin.

Mask #1

Mash the papaya and combine with the pineapple juice (if available) until thoroughly mixed and smooth. Gently pat this onto face and neck. Try to lie down and rest while this mask is doing its job. You may want to place a towel around your head and behind your neck as this mask can be a bit runny. Your face will probably tingle a bit — relax, it just means the ingredients are working properly. Rinse.

The papaya and pineapple contain an enzyme which helps to dissolve and lift away dry skin scales which can, over time, build up on your skin and leave a dull appearance.

Mask #2

Now apply the basic clay mask (see recipe, page 60) using strong sage or rosemary tea in place of the milk, cream, or water to mix with the clay. *If your skin is especially sensitive, use cream as your liquid.* Apply as directed. Dry skin types may want to apply a thin layer of moisturizer first, then proceed with the clay mask. All skin types should apply moisturizer *after* the second mask.

Results: After you've applied your moisturizer, look closely at your face. It should look smoother and more refined. I do this treatment as often as I can when I can get fresh, ripe papaya and pineapple.

HONEY AND WHEAT GERM SOFTENING MASK

1 tablespoon (15 ml) fresh
  honey
1 teaspoon (5 ml) wheat
  germ
1 teaspoon (5 ml) sun-
  flower seed meal

Good for: normal and dry skin
Use: as desired
Follow with: moisturizer, if necessary
Prep time: approximately 5 minutes
Mix with: small bowl and spoon
Store in: Do not store. Mix as needed.
Yields: 1 treatment
Special: Leaves skin soft and moist.

Thoroughly combine all ingredients in a small bowl and allow to set for 1 minute. Pat onto face and neck. Leave on for approximately 30 minutes and rinse after with a very warm damp cloth.

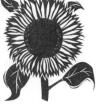

DEEP PORE CLEANSER

1 teaspoon (5 ml) almond
  meal
1 teaspoon (5 ml) sunflower
  seed meal
1 teaspoon (5 ml) ground
  oatmeal
¼ teaspoon (1.25 ml)
  quality vegetable oil
¼ medium-sized ripe
  tomato or 1-inch chunk
  of cucumber, peeled
water

Good for: normal and oily skin
Use: one to two times per week
Follow with: moisturizer
Prep time: 10 to 15 minutes
Mix with: blender, small bowl and spoon
Store in: Do not store. Mix as needed.
Yields: 1 treatment
Special: This recipe can double as a facial
scrub.

Place tomato or cucumber into a blender and add a small amount of water, one tablespoon at most. Blend until smooth. Strain. Combine enough of the vegetable liquid with the meal and oil to form a smooth paste. Spread onto face and neck, allow to dry, rinse.

"PEACHES AND CREAM" GLOW MASK

½ very ripe small peach
   (peeled)
1 tablespoon (15 ml) heavy
   cream

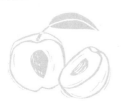

Good for: normal-to-very dry, and sensitive
skin
Use: as desired
Follow with: moisturizer, if necessary
Prep time: approximately 5 minutes
Mix with: mortar and pestle, or small bowl
and fork
Store in: Do not store. Mix as needed.
Yields: 1 treatment
Special: Highly moisturizing and fragrant.

Mash the peach half and combine with cream until smooth. Apply mixture to
face and neck and leave on for 30 minutes while lying down or reclining on a
slant board. Rinse. This mask is as delicious as it is nourishing for your skin.
You may be tempted to mix up a larger quantity (made with milk instead of
cream), add a dab of honey, and drink it for lunch!

   Note: Mask can be runny. You may wish to wrap a towel around your hair
to catch any drips.

APPLESAUCE AND WHEAT GERM MOISTURIZING MASK

1 tablespoon (15 ml) fresh
   applesauce
1 tablespoon (15 ml) raw
   wheat germ
2 teaspoons (10 ml) oil of
   wheat germ, jojoba, or
   sweet almond

Good for: normal and dry skin
Use: as desired
Follow with: moisturizer, if necessary
Prep time: approximately 10 minutes
Mix with: small bowl and spoon
Store in: Do not store. Mix as needed.
Yields: 1 treatment
Special: Leaves skin moist and rosy.

Mix the applesauce and wheat germ thoroughly. Allow mixture to thicken for
5 minutes or until the wheat germ absorbs some of the apple juice. Apply to face
and throat. This is another mask that can be a bit messy. Wrap up your hair
and think pleasant thoughts while your skin drinks in all this moisture. Rinse.
Follow with a nourishing oil facial massage. Simply massage the oil onto your
face and throat in gentle, circular actions for 5 minutes. Towel dry. Your face
should be moist, warm, and glowing!

HONEY MASSAGE MASK

2 to 3 teaspoons (10 to 15 ml) fresh honey
Hair pins or shower cap

Good for: all skin types, especially dehydrated and/or flaky
Use: as desired
Follow with: moisturizer, if necessary
Prep time: two to three minutes
Mix with: n/a
Store in: n/a
Yields: 1 treatment
Special: Softens and moisturizes.

Apply a thin coat of your favorite honey to your entire face and neck. Be sure to pull your hair up and off your face. When honey is spread evenly, it will bead up as water beads up on your car after a shower. Leave on for 15 minutes while you lie down and rest. Your skin will begin to feel very warm and relaxed. Don't fall asleep!

Before rinsing, begin to gently pat your entire face with your fingertips. Make quick tapping motions like you are playing the piano. Do this for about 5 minutes. Rinse with very warm water and a damp cloth.

AVOCADO AND BUTTERMILK MASK

¼ very ripe avocado
Buttermilk

Good for: normal-to-very dry, especially rough or chapped skin
Use: as desired
Follow with: moisturizer, if necessary
Prep time: approximately 5 minutes
Mix with: small bowl and fork
Store in: Do not store. Mix as needed.
Yields: 1 treatment
Special: A larger batch can be made and applied to dry hair to serve as a conditioner for normal and dry hair. Leave on for 30 minutes. Rinse and shampoo out.

Mash together the avocado and just enough buttermilk to form a creamy paste. Apply in upward strokes to face and throat. If possible, lie in the sun to allow the oils of the avocado to warm and penetrate your skin. Rinse after 20 to 30 minutes. Your skin should feel velvety soft.

OATMEAL MASK

4 teaspoons (20 ml)
    ground oatmeal
4 teaspoons (20 ml) milk
    or buttermilk

Good for: all skin types

Use: as desired

Follow with: moisturizer, if necessary

Prep time: approximately 5 minutes

Mix with: small bowl and spoon

Store in: Do not store. Mix as needed.

Yields: 1 treatment

Special: Mask has a slight bleaching effect if used repeatedly. Helps even out a fading tan.

Combine ingredients and allow to thicken for a few minutes. Spread onto face, throat, and chest area. Relax on a slant board if possible, or just recline until dry. Rinse.

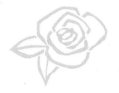

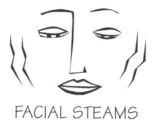

FACIAL STEAMS

An herbal facial steam will soften the skin and allow the pores to perspire and breathe. As the steam penetrates the skin, the various herbs will soften the skin's surface, act as an astringent and/or aid in healing skin lesions. Also, any clogging from dirt or makeup will be loosened for easy removal afterward.

Herbal steams may be used regularly by those with normal, dry, or oily skins. Those of you with sensitive skin or thread veins, however, should abstain.

Always cleanse your skin before steaming.

Preparation: To prepare for a facial steam, boil 3 cups (710 ml) of distilled water. If a recipe calls for vinegar, boil it with the water. Remove from heat and add the herbs to steep, with the lid on the pot, for about 5 minutes. Now, place the pot of herbs in a safe, stable place where you can sit comfortably for 10 minutes. Use a bath towel to create a tent over your head, shoulders, and steaming herb pot. With your eyes closed, breathe deeply and relax as you cleanse your pores with this wonderful, fragrant steam.

Important note: Please allow 8 to 10 inches between the steaming herb pot and your face so you won't risk burning your skin.

After your skin has been "steam cleaned," rinse with tepid water first, then follow with cool splashes. Pat skin until almost dry. Following a facial steam is the ideal time to use a mask and moisturizer so that your skin may benefit from a full treatment. Enjoy!

Special note: If you would like to make up a larger batch of your favorite facial steam mixture to have handy, store the dry ingredients in an airtight zip-seal bag, low tub or

GIFT IDEA

An attractive container to use when giving a freshly made facial steam recipe is a one-quart size, blue or red speckled enameled pot. You can find these in many discount stores or specialty kitchen shops. Make up about ½ cup (118 ml) of the herb mixture from one of the following recipes, put it in a plastic freezer bag, tie with a ribbon, and attach instructions and a measuring spoon. Place this inside the pot (which is to be used to make the facial steam). A nice accompaniment is a bath towel. If you can, choose a towel and pot that are the same color.

jar, or tin, and keep in a dark, cool place. If the recipe calls for added oil or vinegar, add these when you are ready to do a facial steam.

What can you do with the leftover herbal liquid after you have steamed your face? Let it cool and use it to water your plants, strain it and add it to your bath water, or pour the whole mixture onto your compost pile. Don't waste it! *Do not*, however, pour a vinegar solution on your plants.

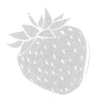

BASIC STEAM

3 cups (710 ml) distilled water

1 teaspoon (5 ml) calendula (marigold)

1 teaspoon (5 ml) chamomile

1 teaspoon (5 ml) raspberry leaves

1 teaspoon (5 ml) peppermint

1 teaspoon (5 ml) strawberry leaves

Good for: all skin types
Use: one to two times per week
Follow with: moisturizer
Prep time: approximately 15 minutes
Mix with: n/a
Store in: Dry ingredients: zip-seal bag, low tub or jar, tin. Keep in cool dark place.
Yields: 1 treatment
Special: Can double as a hair rinse for light brown and blonde/red hair. Strain before using.

Follow this steam up with a mask if you wish, followed by moisturizer.

REFRESHING PORE CLEANSER

3 cups (710 ml) distilled
  water
1 teaspoon (5 ml) yarrow
1 teaspoon (5 ml) sage or
  rosemary
1 teaspoon (5 ml) pepper-
  mint

Good for: normal and oily skin
Use: one to two times per week
Follow with: moisturizer
Prep time: approximately 15 minutes
Mix with: n/a
Store in: Dry ingredients: zip-seal bag, low
tub or jar, tin. Keep in cool dark place.
Yields: 1 treatment

Rinse with tepid water, then cool. Follow this steam with a mask, followed by moisturizer.

pH RESTORER

3 cups (710 ml) distilled
  water
½ (118 ml) cup apple cider
  vinegar
1 teaspoon (5 ml) lavender
  flowers or rosemary
1 teaspoon (5 ml) rose
  petals

Good for: all skin types
Use: one to two times per week
Follow with: moisturizer
Prep time: approximately 15 minutes
Mix with: n/a
Store in: Dry ingredients: zip-seal bag, low
tub or jar, tin. Keep in cool dark place.
Yields: 1 treatment
Special: Softens skin.

This facial steam is particularly good if you wear makeup daily or use soap to cleanse your skin. Most makeup and soap leave an alkaline residue on your skin which leaves it wide open for bacterial infection, pimples, and patchy dryness. Your skin is naturally a bit on the acid side with a pH of approximately 5.5. The vinegar in this steam helps restore your skin's proper pH balance.

After completing this steam, use a mask, followed by moisturizer.

DRY SKIN SAUNA

3 cups (710 ml) distilled
   water
1 teaspoon (5 ml) orange
   peel or orange flowers
1 teaspoon (5 ml) comfrey
   leaves
1 teaspoon (5 ml) elder
   flowers
1 teaspoon (5 ml) sweet
   almond or avocado oil
   (any quality vegetable
   oil will do)

Good for: normal and dry skin
Use: one to two times per week
Follow with: moisturizer
Prep time: approximately 15 minutes
Mix with: n/a
Store in: Dry ingredients: zip-seal bag, low
tub or jar, tin. Keep in cool dark place.
Yields: 1 treatment
Special: Can double as a toner. Strain and
cool. Store and refrigerate. Shake before each
use.

This steam treatment works especially well when followed by a mask and
moisturizer.

WRINKLE CHASER

3 cups (710 ml) distilled
   water
1 tablespoon (15 ml)
   crushed fennel seed
2 drops essential oil of
   rose

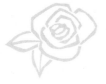

Good for: all skin types, especially dehy-
drated, rough, and chapped
Use: one to two times per week
Follow with: moisturizer
Prep time: 10 to 15 minutes
Mix with: mortar and pestle to crush seeds
Store in: Dry ingredients: zip-seal bag, low
tub or jar, tin. Keep in cool dark place.
Yields: 1 treatment
Special: Soothes and softens skin. This mix-
ture, when strained and cooled, can be used as
a soothing facial splash, mouthwash, or soften-
ing hair rinse. Refrigerate any unused portion.

Follow this treatment up with a mask and moisturizer.

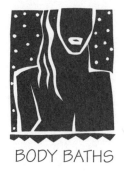

BODY BATHS

Bathing has been an important daily ritual for thousands of years. The bath is not for hygienic purposes alone, but can also be used for pampering the body and spirit. Cleopatra was known for her soothing milk baths and Marie Antoinette for her long, luxurious herbal ones. Healing treatments can be incorporated into the bathing ritual, too. Health spas the world over offer mineral baths in hot springs, sulfur waters, and mud (used to remove impurities from the skin). Various herbal and salt baths are also enjoyable for their fragrant and soothing benefits.

Whether you're interested in soaking your tired, aching muscles and daily tensions away, stimulating your circulation, soothing your dry skin, or enjoying a calming bath laced with essential oil of gardenia, these recipes are sure to please.

Shower fanatics beware: try a few of these tub-tantalizing mixtures and you may become a true bath lover after all!

Special tip: Keep your bath water warm, not hot. Hot water causes your skin to perspire and will not enable your body to absorb the properties of the natural ingredients you choose to include in your bath. Also, the hotter the water, the quicker the essential oils dissipate into the air and lose their qualities, and hot water dehydrates your skin.

GIFT IDEA

Bath salts are an easy-to-make, inexpensive, and warmly welcomed gift. Make up a large batch of the Herbal Bath Salts recipe, enough for about four baths, in a large bowl. Find a decorative tin or jar with a tight-fitting lid and fill with the bath salts. (You might want to put a small muslin bag of rice in the bottom to absorb any moisture that might find its way into the container.) Wrap the container in plain brown paper and gather at the top with ribbon or twine and attach a hand-printed card detailing the instructions.

HERBAL BATH BAG

8-inch x 8-inch square of
   muslin, cheese cloth, or
   foot of an old nylon
   stocking
2 tablespoons (30 ml)
   elder flowers,
   chamomile, lavender,
   lemon balm, or jasmine
1 tablespoon (15 ml)
   raspberry leaves
1 tablespoon (15 ml)
   comfrey leaves
1 tablespoon (15 ml)
   ground oatmeal
String or yarn

Good for: all skin types
Use: as desired
Follow with: moisturize body after bath
Prep time: 10 to 15 minutes
Mix with: n/a
Store in: Several bags could be made and
stored in a zip-seal bag, low tub or jar, or tin.
Yields: 1 treatment
Special: Softens and soothes skin, pleasant
scent.

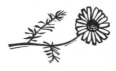

Place herbs and oatmeal in center of cloth or toe of stocking. Gather into a
pouch and tie with a string long enough to hang from the hot water tap in the
tub to allow the running water to flow through. After the tub is full, untie the
bag from the tap and let it float around in the water. Sit back and enjoy!
Discard when finished.

SKIN SOFTENING WASH BAG

¼ cup (59 ml) ground
   oatmeal
¼ cup (59 ml) ground
   sunflower seeds
String or yarn
8-inch x 8-inch square of
   muslin, cheese cloth, or
   foot of an old nylon
   stocking

Good for: normal and dry skin
Use: as desired
Follow with: moisturize body after bath
Prep time: 5 to 10 minutes
Mix with: n/a
Store in: Several bags could be made and
stored in a zip-seal bag, low tub or jar, or tin.
Yields: 1 treatment
Special: Softens and moisturizes skin.

Place ingredients in center of cloth or toe of stocking. Gather into a pouch and
tie with a short string. As you relax in the tub, gently rub your entire body with
the bag, then let it remain in the water releasing its softening properties.
Discard bag when finished.

MILK BATH

½ cup (118 ml) powdered whole milk

1 tablespoon (15 ml) apricot kernel, castor, jojoba, grapeseed, or quality vegetable oil

8 drops essential oil of chamomile, jasmine, lavender, rosemary, or marjoram

Good for: normal and dry skin

Use: as desired

Follow with: moisturize body after bath, if necessary

Prep time: approximately 5 minutes

Mix with: n/a

Store in: Do not store. Make as needed.

Yields: 1 treatment

Special: Leaves skin feeling silky soft.

Pour powdered milk and tablespoon of oil together directly under running bath water. Add essential oil immediately before stepping into tub. Swish with hands to mix. Now relax!

HERBAL BATH SALTS

½ cup (118 ml) baking soda

½ cup (118 ml) sea salt

15 drops essential oil of clary sage, marjoram, lavender, or sandalwood

Good for: all skin types, especially itchy and rashy skin

Use: as desired

Follow with: moisturize body after bath

Prep time: approximately 5 minutes

Mix with: n/a

Store in: A larger amount of bath salts can be made and stored in a zip-seal bag, low tub, jar, or tin.

Yields: 1 treatment

Special: Softens and smoothes rough skin.

Turn on the tap full blast and pour soda and salt mixture into tub. Add essential oil when tub is full and swish water to mix.

SORE MUSCLE SOAK

10-inch x 10-inch square of muslin, cheesecloth, or foot of an old nylon stocking
½ cup (118 ml) Epsom salts
½ cup (118 ml) baking soda
1 tablespoon (15 ml) sage
1 tablespoon (15 ml) marjoram
1 tablespoon (15 ml) chamomile
1 tablespoon (15 ml) pine needles
2 teaspoons (10 ml) lemon balm
2 teaspoons (10 ml) peppermint
10 drops essential oil of eucalyptus, peppermint, or juniper
String or yarn

Good for: all skin types
Use: following exercise, or as desired
Follow with: moisturize body after bath
Prep time: approximately 15 minutes
Mix with: n/a
Store in: Several bags could be made and stored in a zip-seal bag, low tub or jar, or tin.
Yields: 1 treatment
Special: Helps relax tense, sore muscles. The fragrance will soothe frayed nerves.

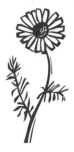

P lace all ingredients in center of cloth and tie into a bag. When adding the essential oil, allow the oil drops to be absorbed by the baking soda before tying the bag. Tie beneath the tap and allow the running water to flow through. When tub is full, remove bag from tap and massage your body with it for a few minutes, then let it float in the tub. Discard after use.

VINEGAR BATH

3 cups (710 ml) apple cider vinegar

½ cup (118 ml) rosemary or juniper berries; either herb may be cut 50/50 with comfrey

Good for: all skin types, except very sensitive

Use: as desired

Follow with: moisturize body after bath

Prep time: 3 to 4 hours

Mix with: n/a

Store in: decorative glass jar or any glass container

Yields: approximately 3 treatments

Special: Soothes and softens itchy skin. Good to use in a foot bath, too.

In a pan, heat vinegar to boiling. Remove from heat and add herbs. Cover and allow to steep for several hours. Strain and store in a pretty container. Use 1 cup per bath. Add liquid to bath while tap is running.

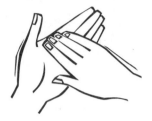

BATH AND MASSAGE OILS

B ath and massage oils are very easy to make at home. You simply need a base oil and any essential oil you desire. I like to use jojoba oil as my base because it does not need refrigeration and will not go rancid. Grapeseed oil makes a great base for massage oil because it is very light and leaves the skin soft, not greasy.

GIFT IDEA

Bath and massage oils are a great treatment for dry skin. In addition, scented oils can be mentally relaxing, stimulating, or can be used to create a sensual mood.

Bath oils make the perfect gift for a friend or loved one who has a particularly stressful lifestyle and enjoys unwinding with a long, luxurious bath. Massage oils (and the accompanying massage) are a great treat for special friends and spouses.

Package oils in blue, green, or brown glass bottles to protect the essential oil from the light. Decorative bottles can be found in antique stores, at flea markets, as well as at bath and gift shops. Make sure the lids fit tightly! Attach a gift card with your personalized message.

NOURISHING OIL

1 tablespoon (15 ml) each of the following oils: sweet almond, virgin olive, avocado, jojoba, apricot kernel, and grapeseed

1,200 international units vitamin E oil (d-alpha tocopherol)

Good for: all skin types, especially normal and dry
Use: as desired
Follow with: moisturize body after bath, if necessary
Oily skin: apply astringent to body, if desired
Prep time: approximately 10 minutes
Mix with: shake before use
Store in: bottle
Yields: approximately 10 treatments, for bath
Special: A good mixture to rub into cuticles, especially if dry and ragged.

Combine ingredients in a bottle. Tightly cap and shake vigorously. Store in refrigerator. For bath, add 2 teaspoons (10 ml) to running water. For massage, use as needed.

FLORAL OIL

¾ cup (118 ml) jojoba oil
½ teaspoon (2.5 ml) essential oil of rose
½ teaspoon (2.5 ml) essential oil of lavender
1 teaspoon (5 ml) essential oil of geranium
¼ teaspoon (1.25 ml) essential oil of ylang-ylang

Good for: normal and dry skin
Use: as desired
Follow with: moisturize body, if necessary
Prep time: 5 to 10 minutes
Mix with: shake before use
Store in: bottle
Yields: approximately 18 treatments, for bath
Special: Softens skin and leaves a romantic floral fragrance upon it.

Mix together the jojoba oil and essential oil, store in a tightly sealed bottle, in a dark place. Add 2 teaspoons (10 ml) oil to bath while tub is filling. For massage, use ½ teaspoon (2.5 ml) essential oil to ½ cup (118 ml) jojoba oil.

To make a glorious floral perfume: Mix the essential oils only, in a beautiful, tiny bottle. Cap tightly and shake well. Apply just a touch on your pulse points: neck, wrists, and behind knees.

STIMULATING HERBAL OIL

¾ cup (118 ml) jojoba oil
2 teaspoons (10 ml) of any
or combination of the
following essential oils:
basil, bay, eucalyptus,
lavender, lemon, lemon-
grass, any of the mints,
pine, rosemary, or tan-
gerine

Good for: all skin types, especially normal and dry
Use: as desired
Follow with: moisturize body after bath, if necessary
Oily skin: apply astringent to body, if desired
Prep time: approximately 10 minutes
Mix with: shake before use
Store in: bottle
Yields: approximately 18 treatments, for bath
Special: A good mixture to rub into cuticles, especially if dry and ragged.

Combine oils, store in a tightly sealed bottle in a dark place. Add 2 teaspoons (10 ml) to running bath water. For massage, use ½ teaspoon (2.5 ml) essential oil to ½ cup (118 ml) jojoba oil.

UPLIFTING OIL

3 teaspoons (15 ml) jojoba
oil
2 drops each, essential
oils of chamomile, pep-
permint, rosemary,
juniper, and eucalyptus

Good for: normal and dry skin
Use: as desired
Follow with: moisturize body, if necessary
Prep time: approximately 5 minutes
Mix with: n/a
Store in: n/a
Yields: 1 treatment
Special: Makes an excellent refreshing and energizing bath oil or deodorizing massage oil for the feet.

Add to bath while tap is running. For foot massage, combine ingredients in a small bowl and have a friend massage your clean, tired feet for 15 minutes, put on socks, and go to bed.

EXOTIC OIL

¾ cup (118 ml) jojoba oil
½ teaspoon (2.5 ml)
    essential oil of sandal-
    wood
½ teaspoon (2.5 ml)
    essential oil of patchouli
½ teaspoon (2.5 ml) musk
    oil, synthetic
¼ teaspoon (1.25 ml)
    essential oil of vetivert

Good for: normal and dry skin
Use: as desired
Follow with: moisturize body, if necessary
Prep time: 5 to 10 minutes
Mix with: shake before use
Store in: bottle
Yields: approximately 18 treatments, for bath
Special: Softens skin and leaves a sensual,
musky fragrance upon it.

Mix together the jojoba oil and essential oil, store in a tightly sealed bottle, in a dark place. Add 2 teaspoons (10 ml) oil to bath while tub is filling. For massage, use ½ teaspoon (2.5 ml) essential oil to ½ cup (118 ml) jojoba oil.
For an exotic perfume: Mix the essential oils only and bottle.

RELAXING OIL

¾ cup (118 ml) jojoba oil
2 teaspoons (10 ml) of any
    of the following essen-
    tial oils: chamomile,
    clary sage, marjoram,
    sandalwood, geranium,
    ylang-ylang, or jasmine

Good for: normal and dry skin
Use: as desired
Follow with: moisturize body, if necessary
Prep time: approximately 5 minutes
Mix with: shake before use
Store in: bottle
Yields: approximately 18 treatments, for bath
Special: Softens skin. Fragrance helps relieve
stress.

Mix together the jojoba oil and essential oil, store in a tightly sealed bottle, in a dark place. Add 2 teaspoons (10 ml) oil to bath while tub is filling. For massage, use ½ teaspoon (2.5 ml) essential oil to ½ cup (118 ml) jojoba oil.

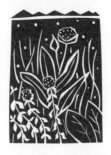

BODY POWDERS

When you think of body powder, the first ingredient that comes to mind is talc, right? Talc is inexpensive but can irritate your lungs and frequently contains traces of arsenic. Besides it's just one of dozens of ingredients you can use as a base powder. Other excellent base powder choices to use alone or in combination include:

- corn flour
- corn starch
- rice flour
- French clay
- powdered calendula flowers
- powdered chamomile flowers

My favorite mixture is one part corn starch, one part arrowroot, and one part powdered calendula flowers. This mixture makes for a very light powder. Sometimes I just use 100% corn starch.

To the base powder, add your favorite essential oil. There you have it — a delightful, all-natural body powder!

GIFT IDEA

Herbal body powders make great Christmas stocking stuffers, Mother's Day, Valentine's Day, or baby shower gifts. Make one of the following recipes and divide it in half or thirds. Find a decorative tin or small powder box that you've stenciled with an ivy or floral design, add the herbal powder so that it fills two-thirds of the container, and add a satin puff or small, fuzzy, fluff brush inside. Top with a bow and label. Some craft stores carry shaker containers, which are always nice for storing body powder. Each recipe will make two to three gifts.

LAVENDER POWDER

¾ pound (340 g) base
 powder mixture
½ pound (227 g) powdered
 lavender flowers
1 to 4 ounces (28 to 113 g)
 powdered rose
 buds/petals (optional)
1 ounce (28 g) powdered
 benzoin gum
½ ounce (14 g) essential
 oil of lavender or rose
 geranium (may mix
 50/50 — makes a nice
 floral fragrance)

Good for: all skin types
Use: as desired
Prep time: 3 days
Mix with: mortar and pestle, flour sifter or
food processor, spoon
Store in: zip-seal bag, box, tin, plastic tub, or
shaker container
Yields: approximately 24 ounces
Special: Makes a light, lovely, old-fashioned
floral-scented body powder.

Combine ingredients in a large bowl or food processor, except the essential oil. Stir with a large spoon or whiz in the food processor for 30 seconds until well blended. Using a mortar and pestle, combine the oil with a few tablespoons of powder until oil is absorbed. Add this mixture to remaining powder and sift together or shake vigorously in a large container with a tight-fitting lid. Whiz for 30 seconds, again, if using a food processor. Store powder in an airtight container and put in a cool, dark place for about 3 days so that the oil can permeate the powder. Use as you would any body powder.

This recipe makes a rather large amount of powder. You may store a portion of the powder in a decorative container for your present use, and the remainder in any airtight container, in a cool, dark place for future use.

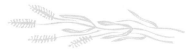

SANDALWOOD POWDER

1 pound (454 g) base pow-
der mixture
1 vanilla bean, chopped into
½-inch pieces
1 ounce (28 g) powdered
benzoin gum
½ ounce (14 g) essential
oil of sandalwood

Good for: all skin types
Use: as desired
Prep time: 3 days
Mix with: mortar and pestle, flour sifter or
food processor, spoon
Store in: zip-seal bag, box, tin, plastic tub, or
shaker container
Yields: approximately 17 ounces (475 g)
Special: Has an earthy, sensual fragrance.

Combine ingredients in a large bowl or food processor, except the essential oil.
Stir with a large spoon or whiz in the food processor for 30 seconds until well
blended. Using a mortar and pestle, combine the oil with a few tablespoons of
powder until oil is absorbed. Add this mixture to remaining powder and sift
together or shake vigorously in a large container with a tight-fitting lid. Whiz for
30 seconds, again, if using a food processor. Store powder in an airtight container and put in a cool, dark place for about 3 days so that the oil can permeate the
powder. Use as you would any body powder.

You may leave the vanilla bean pieces in the powder if you wish, or simply
remove and save them for other uses.

BABY POWDER

½ pound (227 g) base
powder mixture
½ pound (227 g) powdered
chamomile, calendula
(pot marigold), or elder
flowers

Good for: all skin types, especially sensitive
and delicate baby's skin
Use: as desired
Prep time: 10 to 15 minutes
Mix with: large bowl and spoon or food
processor
Store in: zip-seal bag, box, tin, plastic tub, or
shaker container
Yields: approximately 16 ounces (454 g)
Special: Has a very faint, delicate scent. It is a
light, soothing, all-purpose powder.

Combine ingredients thoroughly in a large bowl or food processor. Store.

REFRESHING FOOT POWDER

½ pound (227 g) powder
   base mixture
¼ pound (113 g) powdered
   peppermint
15 drops each essential oil
   of peppermint, eucalyptus, and cajeput
½ ounce (14 g) powdered
   benzoin gum

Good for: all skin types, and especially tired, smelly feet

Use: as desired

Prep time: 3 days

Mix with: mortar and pestle, flour sifter or food processor, spoon

Store in: zip-seal bag, box, tin, plastic tub, or shaker container

Yields: approximately 12 ounces (340 g)

Special: This powder is also nice to use during and after exercise, especially in hot weather.

Combine ingredients in a large bowl or food processor, except the essential oil. Stir with a large spoon or whiz in the food processor for 30 seconds until well blended. Using a mortar and pestle, combine the oil with a few tablespoons of powder until oil is absorbed. Add this mixture to remaining powder and sift together or shake vigorously in a large container with a tight-fitting lid. Whiz for 30 seconds, again, if using a food processor. Store powder in an airtight container and put in a cool, dark place for about 3 days so that the oil can permeate the powder. Use as you would any body powder.

This powder should be sprinkled on clean, dry feet prior to exercise so as to ease friction between toes and shoes and to absorb sweat.

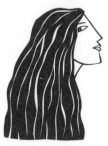

SHAMPOOS, RINSES, AND CONDITIONERS

Most men and women today style their hair to some degree daily. Whether it's simply a quick blow-dry or a complex ritual of moussing, blow-drying, using hot rollers, brushing, applying gel, then topping it all off with hair spray, your hair takes a lot of abuse. There's another factor to consider too...environmental stress. Sunshine, salt water, chlorine, smoking, pollution, and dry office air, all take their toll on your hair's health. Some of you, myself included, have a simple wash-and-wear style, but have a tendency to shampoo quite often, which can strip away your hair's natural oils and leave your crowning glory like straw.

Hair is not meant to take this kind of constant torture. Do your best to find a hair stylist who will cut your hair in a style that it naturally falls into with minimal effort. This will cut down on the number of harsh styling aids you need, shorten your styling time, and it just might save your hair.

GIFT IDEA

Herbal shampoos and conditioners make nice anytime gifts for a special friend.

These recipes can be given in glass or plastic bottles, labeled with instructions, and "wrapped" in a decorative wine bag or gift bag. If you want to give a bottle of Highlight Booster, make sure you tell your friend to refrigerate it. The only recipes I wouldn't give as gifts are the dandruff treatment formulations — unless you and your friend are very close!

If you feel as if you can't live without spray or gels, try your local health food store. There are several natural, nontoxic brands now on the market, and many come in recyclable containers.

The following recipes are quite simple to make and with consistent use will improve the condition of your hair and scalp. The rosemary, chamomile, and calendula rinse recipes will give your highlights a color boost as well as leave your hair very soft and shiny.

HAIR CONDITIONER AND SCALP STIMULATOR

1 teaspoon (5 ml) essential oil of lemongrass

5 teaspoons (25 ml) essential oil of rosemary

3 teaspoons (15 ml) essential oil of lavender

4 teaspoons (20 ml) essential oil of basil

2 teaspoons (10 ml) essential oil of lemon

2 teaspoons (10 ml) essential oil of sandalwood

10 teaspoons (50 ml) jojoba oil

Good for: all hair types
Use: daily or as desired
Follow with: shampoo
Prep time: 5 to 10 minutes
Mix with: shake before use
Store in: dark bottle with dropper or any small, dark, glass bottle
Yields: approximately 14 treatments
Special: Helps stimulate circulation and remove dandruff buildup.

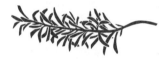

Combine oils and keep tightly closed, in a cool, dark place.

Massage 2 teaspoons (10 ml) into your dry scalp for about 2 to 3 minutes and rub a little onto the ends of your hair. You're not trying to cover your entire head, just the scalp and ends. Wrap your head in plastic or use a shower cap, then wrap again with a very warm, damp towel. Leave on 30 to 45 minutes. Rinse and shampoo.

This conditioner can also be applied in the shower to a warm, wet scalp. Massage, allow to remain in your hair about 3 minutes or longer, rinse, and shampoo. This mixture has a strong fragrance and may tingle slightly — quite invigorating!

BASIC OIL CONDITIONER

¼ cup (59 ml) more or less (depending on length of hair) of one of the following oils: virgin olive, jojoba, sweet almond, or castor

10 drops essential oil of lavender, rosemary, or basil

Good for: normal and dry hair

Use: one time per week

Follow with: shampoo

Prep time: approximately 1 minute

Mix with: n/a

Store in: n/a

Yields: 1 treatment

Special: Excellent for dry, sun-damaged, and chemically treated hair. Leaves hair soft and silky.

Combine the oils and apply to warm, damp (not wet) clean hair. Make sure hair is thoroughly coated. Cover with a plastic bag or shower cap, then cover again with a hot, damp towel. The heat helps the oil to penetrate and condition your hair. Allow to remain on for 30 minutes, then shampoo twice to remove all traces of oil.

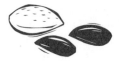

FRAGRANT HAIR SHEEN

Essential oil of rosemary, lavender, or sandalwood

Good for: normal and dry hair

Use: after every shampoo or as desired

Special: Makes hair fragrant and shiny.

In the palm of your hand, place 5 drops essential oil of your choice or 2 drops of each of the oils. Rub palms together and gently pat and scrunch your slightly damp hair. Make sure to distribute oils evenly, paying special attention to ends.

If you set your hair, apply immediately before setting. If you use a blow dryer, apply in the middle of the styling process.

HERBAL SHAMPOO FOR ALL HAIR TYPES

2 cups (473 ml) distilled water

1 tablespoon (15 ml) calendula (pot marigold)

2 teaspoons (10 ml) rosemary

1 tablespoon (15 ml) nettle

2 teaspoons (10 ml) orange peel

2 teaspoons (10 ml) comfrey

2 tablespoons (30 ml) chamomile

½ teaspoon (2.5 ml) essential oil of lavender

1 teaspoon (5 ml) jojoba oil (omit if hair is oily)

½ cup (118 ml) all-natural, gentle baby shampoo

Good for: all hair types
Use: daily or as needed
Follow with: your regular conditioner, Basic Oil Conditioner, Hair Sheen, or Highlight Booster
Prep time: approximately 45 minutes
Mix with: medium-sized bowl and spoon
Store in: bottle
Yields: approximately 40 treatments
Special: Leaves hair shiny and soft. Good baby shampoo, very mild and gentle.

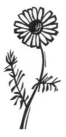

Bring water to a boil and remove from heat. Add the herbs, cover, and allow to steep for 30 minutes. Strain mixture into a medium-sized bowl, add the oils and stir vigorously. Add the shampoo and gently stir until thoroughly mixed. Pour into a labeled bottle and keep refrigerated to preserve the freshness. You may keep a small bottle in the shower with enough shampoo for about one week, if you wish. Use approximately 1 tablespoon (15 ml) per application. This shampoo will not produce mountains of billowy suds as it does not contain strong foaming agents. It cleans gently with minimal sudsing.

Note: Before use, lightly shake shampoo to mix the oil that may separate from the rest of the ingredients.

HERBAL SHAMPOO FOR OILY HAIR

1 tablespoon (15 ml) bur-
dock seeds (crushed) or
leaves
1 tablespoon (15 ml) pep-
permint
1 tablespoon (15 ml) lemon
grass
¼ teaspoon (1.25 ml)
essential oil of clary
sage, tea tree, or rose-
mary
1 tablespoon (15 ml) yarrow
2 cups (473 ml) distilled
water
½ cup (118 ml) all-natural,
baby shampoo

Good for: oily hair
Use: daily or as needed
Follow with: your regular conditioner or
Highlight Booster
Prep time: approximately 45 minutes
Mix with: medium-sized bowl and spoon
Store in: bottle
Yields: approximately 40 treatments
Special: Leaves hair soft and shiny and in
good condition. In a pinch, can double as a
face wash.

Bring water to a boil and remove from heat. Add the herbs, cover, and allow
to steep for 30 minutes. Strain mixture into a medium-sized bowl, add the oil
and stir vigorously. Add the shampoo and gently stir until thoroughly mixed.
Pour into a labeled bottle and keep refrigerated to preserve the freshness of the
herbal liquid. You may keep a small bottle in the shower with enough shampoo
for about a week, if you wish. Use approximately 1 tablespoon (15 ml) per application.

HIGHLIGHT BOOSTERS

Brown/black hair — sage, rosemary, quassia chips, crushed walnut hulls

Blonde hair — chamomile, crushed rhubarb root

Red hair — calendula (pot marigold)

3 cups (710 ml) distilled or spring water

Good for: Rosemary, chamomile, and calendula can be used on any type of hair. The other herbs are somewhat astringent, and best used on hair that is normal or oily. If necessary, follow the rinse with a leave-in conditioner to counteract the drying effect of these herbs.

Use: daily or as needed

Follow with: conditioner, if necessary

Prep time: 35 to 40 minutes

Mix with: spoon

Store in: bottle

Yields: 3 to 5 treatments

Bring water to a boil and remove from heat. Add 3 heaping tablespoons (44 to 59 ml) of the herb(s) of your choice, stir, cover, and allow to steep for 30 minutes. Strain, label, and store in a quart-size plastic bottle. Keep refrigerated.

Shampoo hair, rinse. Squeeze out excess water from hair, then generously pour herbal liquid until hair is saturated. Squeeze out excess.

If you'd like to make a mild shampoo, cut your usual shampoo 50/50 with the rinse of your choice and shampoo as usual. Mild mixture does not need to be refrigerated if used within two weeks.

Note: Use dark towels when drying hair as the herbal liquid will stain lighter-colored ones.

RINSE TO DARKEN GRAY HAIR

1 ounce (28 g) sage
2 ounces (57 g) black
   walnut hulls
2 tablespoons (30 ml)
   regular loose tea (2
   teabags will do fine)
1 ounce (28 g) rosemary
1 ounce (28 g) nettle
2 teaspoons (10 ml) jojoba,
   castor, sweet almond,
   or virgin olive oil
8 cups (1.9 liters) distilled
   or spring water
rubber or latex gloves

Good for: medium-to-dark gray, light-to-dark brown and auburn hair; for all hair types except very dry and/or chemically treated

Use: daily for 2 weeks, then as desired

Follow with: good quality conditioner

Prep time: approximately 4 hours

Mix with: shake before use

Store in: quart-sized bottles

Yields: approximately 16 treatments

Special: Leaves hair shiny and soft.

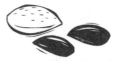

Boil water and remove from heat. Add herbs, cover, and steep for 3 to 4 hours. Strain, add oil, and store in refrigerator. Discard any remaining liquid after 3 weeks. Shampoo as usual and rinse. Before you begin this procedure, put on your gloves. This rinse will stain hands and nails dark brown. Shake bottle thoroughly, and apply about ½ cup (118 ml) of the herbal liquid and massage into scalp and hair for about 1 minute. Squeeze out excess and towel dry hair. Make sure you use a dark towel as this mixture *will stain* lighter-colored ones.

I usually get on my knees and hang my head over the bath tub when I do this rinse. If it splatters in the tub or on your face, it will wipe off.

I also wash my hair using 1 tablespoon (15 ml) of a mixture of ¼ cup (59 ml) baby shampoo and ¼ cup (59 ml) of this dark rinse. No gloves necessary for this treatment. I use it daily and doctor it with ¼ teaspoon (1.25 ml) each essential oil of lavender and rosemary and a few drops of jojoba oil. Discard this mixture after 2 weeks.

Note: The more porous your hair, the more quickly the hair strands will absorb the color. Thick, coarse hair will be quite resistant to taking any herbal color. Everyone's hair is different. Some gray may turn light brown, dark blonde, or medium-to-dark brown.

Anti-Dandruff Treatments

If you begin to see those pesky white flakes in your hair or on your shoulders, it's best to avoid or at least minimize the use of hair gels and sprays, hot blow dryers, harsh shampoos, perms, colors, and straighteners. These can cause a flaky, dry scalp which can imitate dandruff. True dandruff itches and can be a result of hormonal disturbances, faulty diet, emotional stress, or an infection. For a very stubborn case of dandruff, consult your physician; otherwise, the recipes below work quite well.

ROSEMARY SOFTENING RINSE

½ cup (118 ml) rosemary
1 teaspoon (5 ml) borax
4 cups (946 ml) distilled
    or spring water

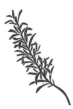

Good for: all hair types, especially lifeless, dull, and flaky
Use: daily or as desired
Follow with: Fragrant Hair Sheen, if desired
Prep time: approximately 2 hours
Mix with: spoon
Store in: bottle
Yields: 4 to 8 rinses, depending on length of hair
Special: Gives hair lustre and body.

Bring water to a boil and remove from heat. Add herbs and borax, stir, cover, and steep for approximately 2 hours. Strain, bottle, and use within 10 days or discard. Use as the final rinse after shampooing and conditioning. Do not rinse out. May stain light-colored towels. Use approximately ½ to 1 cup (118 to 237 ml) per application.

HERBAL VINEGAR INFUSION

2 cups (473 ml) distilled or
  spring water
½ cup (118 ml) apple cider
  vinegar
4 tablespoons (59 ml)
  rosemary
1 tablespoon (15 ml) nettle
10 drops essential oil of
  tea tree, clary sage, or
  rosemary

Good for: all hair types, except very dry
Use: daily or as needed
Follow with: Fragrant Hair Sheen, if desired,
or leave-in conditioner
Prep time: approximately 2 hours
Mix with: shake before use
Store in: bottle
Yields: approximately 10 treatments
Special: Helps to relieve an itchy scalp and
restores pH balance.

Bring the water and vinegar to a boil. Remove from heat. Add herbs, cover, and steep for about 2 hours. Strain, add essential oil, and bottle. No need to refrigerate. Shampoo hair and rinse, or, if not shampooing, wet hair and squeeze out excess. Apply approximately ¼ cup (59 ml) to wet scalp and gently massage for 2 to 3 minutes. Rinse with cool water. Try to use daily until itching and flaking stops.

LIP BALM

Your lips, unlike the rest of your skin, do not contain any sebaceous glands (oil glands) or sweat glands to keep them moisturized and lubricated. Thus, many of you, myself included, constantly slather them in lipsticks and balms of various kinds, in an attempt to prevent drying and cracking.

As you may know, many brands of lipsticks tend to be drying instead of moisturizing. Some can cause your lips to flake and peel and become unsightly. I have yet to see an "all-day formula" that lasts past midmorning. But take heart; I have created a very moisturizing formula that you can make with or without color.

The colorless version can be worn alone or as a base or top coat with your favorite lipstick.

The color version contains no drying chemicals, mica or fish scales for shimmer, or that strange lipstick metallic taste which can linger in your mouth for hours and looks great alone. It's just your basic, nourishing lip balm with a hint of gloss. It even smells and tastes like honey. Your children can use it too!

GIFT IDEA

There's a company called Lavender Lane (see Appendix) which sells .25 ounce (7.5 ml) lip balm jars. They come in three different styles and are the perfect container to hold all the flavors and colors of lip balm you wish to make.

Lip treatments make great stocking stuffers at Christmas, an added treat to a college-bound student's "care package," or a real necessity for someone going skiing or vacationing in the tropics. School-age children can carry a container in their purse or jacket pocket.

LIP BALM/GLOSS

5 to 6 tablespoons (75 to 90 ml) sweet almond, jojoba, castor, or quality vegetable oil

1 tablespoon (15 ml) beeswax

2 teaspoons (10 ml) pure honey

10 drops essential oil of spearmint or peppermint for a sweet taste, or tea tree for treatment of cold sores and chapped, flaky lips (optional)

½ tube favorite colored moisturizing lipstick (optional)

Good for: everyone
Use: as desired
Prep time: 30 to 40 minutes
Mix with: whisk or spoon
Store in: small glass or plastic cosmetic jars or any small container
Yields: approximately 3 ounces (90 ml)
Special: Makes a rich and soothing lip treatment.

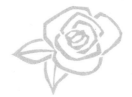

Melt together the oil and beeswax, in a small saucepan over low heat, or in a double boiler just until wax is melted. Use the larger amount of oil if you want a thinner, glossier consistency. Remove from heat. Add honey and blend mixture thoroughly.

If you would like to add color to your gloss, add the piece of lipstick now, while the mixture is still hot. I usually divide the mixture into two containers; one for a colorless gloss and one for a rich cinnamon color gloss.

Stir the mixture(s) occasionally as it cools to prevent separation. It should have the consistency of petroleum jelly when ready.

If you choose to add an essential oil to your lip treatment, add it after the gloss has almost cooled and stir thoroughly.

FLAVORED LIP BALM

2 teaspoons (10 ml)
  beeswax
7–8 teaspoons (35 ml)
  sweet almond, castor,
  jojoba, or quality veg-
  etable oil
1 teaspoon (5 ml) honey
5 drops essential oil of
  lemon, lime, orange, tangerine, peppermint, or
  apple blossom
small piece of moisturizing
  lipstick (optional)

Good for: everyone, especially children
Use: as desired
Prep time: 20 to 30 minutes
Mix with: whisk or spoon
Store in: small glass or plastic lip balm jars
Yields: approximately 1½ ounces (45 ml)
Special: Great for chapped lips. Can double as
a cuticle cream.

Melt together the oil and beeswax, in a small saucepan over low heat, or in a double boiler just until wax is melted. Use the larger amount of oil if you want a thinner, glossier consistency. Remove from heat. Add honey and blend mixture thoroughly. If you would like to add color to your lip balm, add the small piece of lipstick now, while the mixture is still hot. Stir mixture occasionally as it cools to prevent separation. When the mixture is almost cooled, add the essential oil of choice and stir thoroughly. Store in a small container.

This lip balm should have the consistency of paste wax when ready.

Note: Synthetic flavoring oils, such as apple, apricot, cherry, peach, raspberry, or vanilla, can also be used. Children really like these flavors.

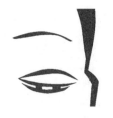

EYE TREATMENTS

It's said that the eyes are the windows to the soul. I don't know if this saying is true or not, but I do know that if you stay up nights with an infant, look at a computer screen all day, party all night, sleep with your eyes squished into a pillow, spend time around smokers or in dry office air, have allergies, get makeup remover in your eyes, or forget to remove your mascara, your "windows" are going to look puffy, bloodshot, irritated, or have dark circles beneath them. They may even sting and tear.

To help soothe, brighten, and refresh red and weary eyes, I've designed the following recipes and suggestions.

Your eyes are your most expressive features — do your best to pamper them. And always make sure to get plenty of sleep. This is the best "eye treatment" of all!

NIGHTTIME EYE MOISTURIZER

Few drops jojoba, grape-seed, sweet almond, or apricot kernel oil

Good for: normal and dry skin
Use: daily
Store in: All oils should be kept in refrigerator, except jojoba.
Special: Highly moisturizing and refreshing if the oil is cold.

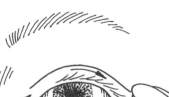
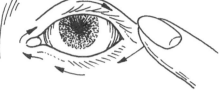

*C*leanse and tone your face and leave slightly damp. Pour a few drops of oil into the palm of your hand. Dip your ring finger into the oil and gently pat the oil around (not directly on) your eye in this fashion: Begin at the outer corner and slowly move beneath your eye toward the inner corner, then onto the very upper portion of the lid and back out to the outer corner.

Do this several times, then pat off any excess oil. Try to leave a light film of oil on your skin.

The reason for not applying the oil directly onto the lid and lashes is that if any of the oil were to get into your eye, it could clog your tear ducts and cause puffiness (which we're trying to avoid!). The delicate eye area will draw the moisture it needs from the surrounding moisturized tissue.

To help relieve puffiness and dark circles, apply any of the following to your eyes while resting for 15 minutes:

- ◆ cold, damp tea bags or cotton squares soaked in chilled tea of catnip, chamomile, elder flower, eyebright, fennel, lavender, orange pekoe or regular tea
- ◆ thin slices of cold cucumber or potato
- ◆ cold witch hazel-soaked pads

EYE RINSE

2 tablespoons (30 ml) eye-bright, chamomile, or crushed fennel seeds
1 cup (237 ml) distilled water

Good for: tired and bloodshot eyes
Use: as desired
Prep time: approximately 1 hour
Mix with: shake before use
Store in: sterilized bottle or spritzer
Yields: approximately 8 ounces
Special: Very refreshing.

*B*ring water to a boil and remove from heat. Add herb, cover, and steep for about 1 hour. Strain, store, and refrigerate. To use, either splash opened eyes with the brew or mist eyes lightly. Feels so wonderful when the liquid is very cold. Discard remaining mixture after 10 days.

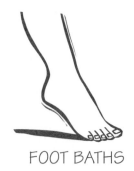

FOOT BATHS

Your feet were designed to be strong yet flexible, support your weight, and provide leverage while walking. There are a few of you who think feet are a beautiful, sensuous part of the body. I have a feeling, though, that most of you would rather hide your tootsies than show them off!

As an aesthetician, I have heard many complaints from clients regarding their feet: "They constantly hurt." "My callouses are so thick, I could cut them with a knife." "My toenails are getting narrow, thick, and ugly." "I'm constantly battling foot odor." Most of these problems are easily rectified.

I usually begin by asking an important question: What kind of shoes do you wear? Many women's shoes are designed purely for fashion, not comfort. They are pointy, high-heeled, too narrow, and frequently too small. At least most men's shoes are generally flat and reasonably comfortable. Ill-fitting footwear can cause a myriad of foot problems. You may find that purchasing properly fitting, attractive, "sensible" shoes will solve problems with chronic achiness and tiredness. Foot odor can usually be remedied by wearing natural fiber socks and shoes that breathe.

> **GIFT IDEA**
>
> A good recipe to give a family member or close friend as a gift is the Foot Scrub recipe, packaged dry. Double or triple the recipe and package it in a decorative tin or jar, or store it in a zip-seal bag and put inside a cardboard or wooden box. You could stencil or draw some footprints on the box for an artistic touch. Whatever packaging you choose, be sure to label the container and include directions for use inside. A nice accompaniment would be a ¼ ounce (7.5 ml) bottle of lemon or peppermint essential oil either placed inside the container or attached to the outside with a ribbon.

If you have other foot problems, such as bunions, hammer toe, fallen arches, excessive perspiration and odor, see a podiatrist, as he/she specializes in foot disorders.

In the meantime, treat your feet with the following recipes designed to bring relief to tired, rough, itchy, dry, thickened, abused, neglected, and odoriferous dogs. Many of the recipes require the use of a foot tub. These can be purchased for a few dollars from your local grocery or hardware store. What you're looking for is essentially a plastic dishpan approximately 5 inches (13 cm) deep, 12 inches (31 cm) wide, and 12 to 23 inches (31 to 59 cm) long. If you really want to pamper your feet, you may want to consider a foot tub with mini-Jacuzzi action and vibrating foot pads. Available from most department stores and better drug stores, this is a decidedly more indulgent, and expensive, option.

Special tips: *Foot rollers* are available in health food stores and other shops that sell bath products. They are wonderful for relieving sore, tired, tense feet. I prefer the wooden ones that have ridges from one end to the other. They are more stimulating than the smooth ones!

Foot massage, what a luxury to receive! Massage your loved one's clean feet with a mixture of coconut, castor, grapeseed, or your favorite oil, and a few drops of your favorite essential oil. Then let him or her massage your feet. A great way to spend the evening with your "sole mate"!

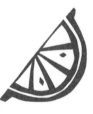

FOOT SCRUB

¼ cup (59 ml) ground oatmeal
¼ cup (59 ml) cornmeal
1 tablespoon (15 ml) sea or table salt
Essential oil of lemon or peppermint
Spring or tap water

Good for: rough, dry, calloused feet
Use: daily or as needed
Follow with: moisturizer
Prep time: 5 to 10 minutes
Mix with: spoon and small bowl
Store in: A large batch of the dry mix could be made, stored in a zip-seal bag, low tub/jar, or tin and kept in the bathroom.
Yields: 1 treatment
Special: Leaves feet feeling soft, smooth, tingly, and the body refreshed.

Combine the dry ingredients with enough water to form a creamy, gritty paste. Add a few drops of essential oil and stir again. Sit on the edge of the bathtub or bench in the shower and massage feet with mixture. *Really scrub* all those rough areas and between toes. I find this quite invigorating. Rinse and dry. Apply a thick moisturizing cream mixed with a few drops of either essential oil.

Note: Make sure to clean the bathtub after this procedure as the scrub could clog the drain.

FOOT SOOTHER

Foot tub
1 cup (237 ml) apple cider
   vinegar
2 tablespoons (30 ml)
   glycerin

Good for: dry and itchy feet
Use: daily or as desired
Follow with: moisturizer and foot powder
Prep time: approximately 5 minutes
Mix with: swish feet in tub to mix ingredients
Store in: Do not store. Mix as needed.
Yields: 1 treatment
Special: Helps to relieve athlete's foot symptoms.

Place ingredients into your foot tub and enough water, warm or cold, to cover your feet and ankles. Soak for 15 to 20 minutes. Pat dry.

FOOT REFRESHER

Foot tub
Marbles
5 to 10 drops of essential
   oil of lemon, lavender,
   camphor, peppermint,
   rosemary, juniper, or
   eucalyptus
½ cup (118 ml) sea salt
   (table salt is fine)

Good for: tired and aching feet
Use: daily or as desired
Follow with: moisturizer
Prep time: 5 to 10 minutes
Mix with: swish feet in tub
Store in: Do not store. Mix as needed.
Yields: 1 treatment
Special: Especially good for athletes or people who are on their feet all day.

To a tub of very hot or very cold water, add oil of choice and salt. Make sure there's enough water to cover ankles. Now put in enough marbles to almost cover the bottom of the tub where your feet are resting. Soak feet for 15 to 20 minutes while gently rolling them back and forth over the marbles. Occasionally, grasp and release marbles with toes. This action stretches and relaxes the feet. Roughly rub feet dry and apply a soothing lotion mixed with a few drops of one of the above-mentioned essential oils.

FOOT DEODORIZER

Foot tub
6 quarts (5.7 litres) water
5 to 10 drops essential oil
   of rosemary, lavender,
   peppermint, or eucalyptus
½ cup (118 ml) baking soda
½ cup (118 ml) sage, lavender, peppermint, or
   rosemary

Good for: foot odor
Use: daily or as needed
Follow with: foot powder
Prep time: approximately 40 minutes
Mix with: swish feet in tub
Store in: Do not store. Mix as needed.
Yields: 1 treatment
Special: Leaves feet feeling soft.

Boil 6 quarts (5.7 litres) water, remove from heat, and add herb. Cover and steep 30 minutes. Strain. Add the herbal infusion, baking soda, and essential oil to foot bath and swish. Soak feet for approximately 15 to 20 minutes. Towel dry.

CALLOUS REMOVER

Foot tub
½ cup (118 ml) sea salt
   (table salt is fine)
½ cup (118 ml) baking soda
Pumice stone or pedi-wand
   (available in health food
   stores or beauty supply
   houses)

Good for: rough, calloused feet
Use: daily or as needed
Follow with: heavy moisturizer and socks
Prep time: 5 to 10 minutes
Mix with: swish feet in tub
Store in: Do not store. Mix as needed.
Yields: 1 treatment
Special: Leaves feet feeling soft and smooth.

Thoroughly dissolve the baking soda and salt in your tub of hot water. Soak feet for 20 minutes, or longer, if calluses are very thick. Remove feet from water, and while still wet, gently scrub calluses with pumice stone or the rough side of a pedi-wand. When you see the loose skin building up on the scrubbing tool, dip it and your foot into the solution, rinse, and begin again if necessary. Roughly rub feet dry and apply a thick cream or non-petroleum jelly. Now put on cotton socks. This will continue to soften your feet throughout the day or overnight. This procedure can also be done in the bathtub after your feet have become soft. I usually bathe, mask, and smooth my feet during a bath. A great time-saver in my busy schedule.

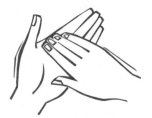

HAND AND NAIL TREATMENTS

Next time you're at a social function, take a glance at the hands of several people. Can you tell, just by looking at their hands, what kind of work they do? A mechanic's hands and nails will frequently be grease-stained. An accountant, attorney, or secretary's will be smooth and soft. A full-time mother with several children and a small garden will probably have dry skin and cuticles, and a carpenter, brick mason, or farmer may have rough, cracked, suntanned hands with hard fingernails and thick callouses.

We tend to pay so much attention to our face and hair, but often neglect one of our most expressive features, our hands. They are constantly exposed to the elements: sun, wind, heat, cold, harsh cleansers, dirt, grease, etc., and are one of the first places on our body to show age.

You can fight the ravages of time and the elements by remembering to take a few important steps each day. Apply moisturizer frequently, wear rubber gloves when hands will be exposed to water or cleansers, and wear garden gloves when working outdoors. Don't forget to apply a sunscreen with a SPF-15 whenever you're in the sun. Sun damage can result in premature aging of the skin, blotchiness, dryness and "liver spots."

The recipes below will help to soften and protect your hands and nails.

GIFT IDEA

A small basket of hand and nail care products makes the perfect gift for someone who works with their hands or frequently exposes them to the elements. Fill a basket with a jar of the Hand and Nail Butter, a 10-inch x 10-inch piece of soft cotton flannel (hem the edges first), nail file, clippers, cuticle scissors, and a nail buffer. Add or subtract any items you wish to personalize the gift. A pair of white cotton gloves for an overnight treatment and a tube of sunscreen make a nice accompaniment.

Attach instructions for the Hand and Nail Butter.

HAND AND NAIL BUTTER

2 tablespoons (30 ml)
beeswax

2 tablespoons (30 ml)
cocoa butter

4 tablespoons (59 ml)
grapeseed or jojoba oil

1 tablespoon (15 ml) anhydrous lanolin

20 drops essential oil of
rose, carrot seed, rose-
mary, geranium, or san-
dalwood (optional)

Good for: everyone, especially those with dry, rough, chapped hands and cuticles

Use: daily or as desired

Follow with: n/a

Prep time: approximately 30 minutes

Mix with: whisk or spoon

Store in: low tub or jar

Yields: approximately 27 treatments

Special: Very rich and moisturizing. Smells like chocolate if left unscented.

In a small saucepan or double boiler, warm all ingredients, except essential oil, until wax is melted. Remove from heat and stir occasionally until almost cool, add essential oil, if desired, stir again, and store. Use approximately 1 teaspoon (5 ml) per application as a hand cream or nail and cuticle treatment. Can use on hands and feet as overnight intensive treatment. Wear gloves or socks. Use within 3 to 4 months. Requires no refrigeration.

Note: This recipe may harden in cold weather, but will soften upon skin contact.

Nail and cuticle treatment: Soak clean hands in a bowl of warm water for 2 minutes. Pat dry. Apply a dab of "Butter" onto the base of each nail and massage in. Using a small piece of cotton flannel, gently push cuticles back and lightly buff nails with the cloth. Leaves fingertips soft and smooth.

Naturally shiny nail treatment: Apply the "Butter" the same as for the nail and cuticle treatment above, but use a nail buffer to gently polish nails to a soft sheen. Don't rub so hard that your nails burn. Do this once a week.

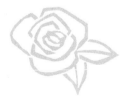

CASTOR OIL SOAK

4 to 5 tablespoons (60 to 75 ml) castor oil
10 drops essential oil of sandalwood

Good for: dry, brittle, weak nails and cuticles
Use: three times per week
Follow with: moisturizer
Prep time: 1 to 2 minutes
Mix with: fingers
Store in: low tub/jar or small bowl
Yields: 3 treatments
Special: Helps strengthen nails and relieve drying and cracking of cuticles.

In a small bowl, combine oils. Soak clean fingertips for 5 to 10 minutes. Using a soft cloth, push back cuticles and lightly buff nails. Use the same mixture for 3 treatments. Keep covered and refrigerate.

SKIN LIGHTENING HAND PACK

2 tablespoons (30 ml) ground oatmeal
1 tablespoon (15 ml) plain yogurt
1 teaspoon (5 ml) any quality oil
2 teaspoons (10 ml) fresh pineapple, lemon, or strawberry juice

Good for: sun-damaged, dry, unevenly colored hands
Use: two times per week
Follow with: moisturizer or SPF-15 sunscreen
Prep time: 5 to 10 minutes
Mix with: spoon and small bowl
Store in: Do not store. Mix as needed.
Yields: 1 treatment
Special: Leaves hands soft and smooth.

Combine ingredients to form a paste and allow to thicken for 1 minute. If too thick, add a bit of water to thin slightly. Apply mixture to back of hands and allow to dry for 15 to 30 minutes. Rinse with cool water. Pat almost dry and apply a good moisturizer or sunscreen.

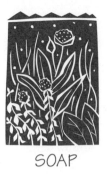

SOAP

Most soaps on the market today are highly alkaline and can strip your skin of its natural oils, leaving it dry, tight, and prone to eczema. I don't generally recommend that anyone use soap on their face and neck unless they have extremely oily skin. Even then, only a very gentle, pH-balanced soap should be used.

I am well aware that there are those of you who swear by soap. You've used it all your life, every day, from head to toe, and even to wash your hair. It makes you feel clean. All I can say is, you must have tough skin. If I engaged in this practice, my skin would resemble the look and feel of a dried prune, shoe leather, or some ghastly looking, wrinkled, desert-dwelling creature!

Old habits are hard to break, so I've developed this recipe for you diehard soap fans. At least it is a healthy departure from your usual brand.

GIFT IDEA

Know anyone who tends a garden, has small children, or an occupation that requires lots of hand-washing? What a great gift these soap balls would be. They're so much more gentle to your skin than regular soap.

Double the recipe and make 5 medium-sized or 10 small soap balls and place them inside a nice pottery or wooden bowl. Place the bowl in a decorative gift bag lined with tissue paper or craft straw. Attach a note card describing the softening ingredients in the soap and a reminder not to leave the soap in the shower or standing water because it will melt.

SUPER-FATTED, ALL-PURPOSE
HERBAL BODY SOAP BALLS

Two 3.5 ounce (10.5 ml)
  bars unscented castile
  soap or pure glycerine
  soap, grated
2 tablespoons (30 ml)
  ground oatmeal or corn-
  meal
1 tablespoon (15 ml)
  crushed lavender, rose-
  mary or peppermint (or
  use your favorite herb
  for your skin type)
10 drops favorite essential
  oil
1 tablespoon (15 ml) anhydrous lanolin
1 tablespoon (15 ml) sweet
  almond, castor, jojoba,
  or quality vegetable oil
Oil for hands

Good for: normal and oily skin
Use: daily
Follow with: toner and/or moisturizer
Prep time: approximately 45 minutes
Mix with: spoon
Store in: wax paper wrap, place in cool, dry area
Yields: 2 to 3 medium-sized balls or 2 round cakes
Special: Leaves skin feeling soft and clean.

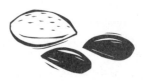

Melt grated soap, lanolin, and oil over low heat in a small saucepan or double boiler until the mixture is a very soft, mushy consistency. Stir occasionally while melting. Remove from heat and stir in remaining ingredients.

While soap mixture is still hot, oil your hands, and form the soap into balls. You can make any size you like, but I think the size of a lime is a good size to handle. Place the balls on wax paper to cool. Use this soap as you would regular soap, but do not leave it in a puddle in the shower as it will melt. If you prefer round cakes of soap to balls, this recipe will yield approximately 2 cakes.

DENTIFRICES AND MOUTHWASHES

Most commercial tooth-pastes on the market today contain harsh abrasives, which, over the years, wear down tooth enamel and gum tissue. Many also contain saccharin, sugar, and detergents. Most mouthwashes aren't any better. They're colored with artificial dyes and flavor, contain alcohol, and harsh chemicals. Why submit your teeth and gums to such torture? Try a gentle, natural approach by using the following recipes.

Note: If you have chronic bad breath or dental problems, see your dentist.

GIFT IDEA

To give a lovely basket of just dental hygiene products is like saying, in a not-so-subtle way, "Gee, your breath smells horrible . . . but I hope you have a nice day, anyway." This is not advisable! It would be better to give a "sampler basket." By this I mean, combine a body powder and massage oil with a hand cream and an herbal mouthwash. This way your friend can sample the variety of herbal products you make, without being offended.

ANTISEPTIC MOUTHWASH AND GARGLE

6 ounces (180 ml) of
  water
3 to 4 drops essential oil
  of clove or tea tree

Good for: sore, bleeding gums, cold sores in the mouth, and sore throat
Use: daily or as needed
Prep time: approximately 1 minute
Mix with: spoon
Store in: Do not store. Mix as needed.
Yields: 1 treatment
Special: Mouth should feel cool and possibly a bit numb.

Stir water and oil together in a small glass. Swish in your mouth and gargle for 30 seconds, then spit out. Repeat 1 to 2 more times. May use this mixture throughout the day to help relieve sore throat and cold sores if necessary.

SODA/SALT PASTE

1 teaspoon (5 ml) baking soda or finely ground sea salt
1 drop essential oil of peppermint, clove, cinnamon, or spearmint
Few drops of water

Good for: everyone
Use: daily
Follow with: water rinse or mouthwash
Prep time: 1 to 2 minutes
Mix with: toothbrush and small bowl
Store in: Do not store. Mix as needed.
Yields: 1 treatment
Special: Leaves mouth feeling clean and fresh. Cinnamon oil may irritate sensitive gums and tongue.

Combine ingredients in a tiny bowl and mix thoroughly until a smooth, thick paste forms. Don't make it too runny or it won't stay on your toothbrush. Use as you would your regular toothpaste.

STRAWBERRY BRIGHTENER

1 medium-sized ripe strawberry

Good for: everyone, especially those with stained teeth
Use: daily
Follow with: water rinse or mouthwash
Prep time: approximately 1 minute
Mix with: mash fruit with mortar and pestle
Store in: n/a
Yields: 1 treatment
Special: Leaves mouth feeling clean and wonderful tasting.

Mash strawberry into a pulp. Dip your brush into the liquid and brush normally. Strawberries have a slight bleaching effect and help to rid the teeth of tea, coffee, and cigarette stains. A strawberry is much safer to use than lemon juice, which is too acidic.

TOOTH TWIG

3-inch to 4-inch twig from a sweet gum or flowering dogwood tree (twig must be "just cut" from the tree)

Good for: everyone
Use: daily
Follow with: water rinse or mouthwash
Prep time: 2 to 3 minutes
Yields: 1 treatment
Special: This is definitely a recyclable toothbrush, about as natural as they come!

Peel the twig and chew on the end until it is frayed and soft. It should taste slightly sweet. Now gently rub your teeth and gums. This is a very "old fashioned" way of brushing your teeth, but it's effective. The twig can also be dipped in water and soda, if you desire.

HERBAL MOUTHWASH

2 cups (473 ml) distilled water
2 tablespoons (30 ml) peppermint, spearmint, or rosemary
10 drops tincture of benzoin or 1 teaspoon (5 ml) tincture of myrrh

Good for: everyone, especially those with bad breath, sore and/or bleeding gums
Use: daily
Prep time: approximately 8 hours or overnight
Mix with: shake before use
Store in: bottle
Yields: approximately 16 rinses
Special: Leaves mouth feeling cool and tingly.

Boil water and remove from heat. Add herb of choice, cover, and steep for about 8 hours or overnight. After the liquid has cooled, you can put the pot in the refrigerator to steep overnight, if you wish. Strain, add either tincture (acts as a preservative and antiseptic), and bottle. Use approximately 2 tablespoons (30 ml) per use.

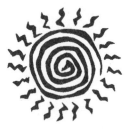

SUNTANNING CREAM, SUNSCREEN, AND AFTER-SUN RELIEF

Light to moderate exposure to the sun makes us feel good, it helps the body manufacture vitamin D, gives us energy after a long, cold winter, it warms the soul, and leaves a rosy-golden glow upon the skin. On the flipside, overexposure dries our skin, causes wrinkles, blotchiness, and premature aging, and increasingly, leads to skin cancer.

In my opinion, 10 to 20 minutes of sun exposure each day, (without sunscreen), *before* 10:30 A.M. or *after* 4:30 P.M., is good for your physical health as well as your emotional well-being. There are many that disagree with me, but I feel that with such a light exposure to the sun, the benefits outweigh any possible harm.

However, if you are going to be in the sun for a longer period of time, *by all means* apply a good sunscreen. This is especially important if you're going to be on or near water, or even relaxing on a sandy beach. Water and sand can reflect the sun's powerful rays, further increasing the chances of overexposure and skin damage. I always wear a sunscreen with at least a SPF-15. You may need an even stronger one, depending on your skin type.

GIFT IDEA

Know any sun worshippers? Everyone does! By March 1, they're outside trying to get a jump on their summer tan, even if there's still snow on the ground! Many of these people aren't too keen on using sunscreen, either, but I'm sure they would appreciate a bottle of your freshly made, low SPF Sunscreen Body Oil.

Fill an 8-ounce (240 ml) plastic squeeze bottle with your wonderful-smelling creation, apply a decorative label, and tie a piece of twine with a couple of seashells attached to each end, around the top.

If you want to preserve the beauty of your skin for years to come and help prevent skin cancer, do not spend excess time in the sun, unprotected.

DURING AND AFTER-SUN BODY LOTION

4 tablespoons (59 ml) aloe
   vera gel
2 tablespoons (30 ml)
   chamomile, comfrey, or
   fennel tea
2 tablespoons (30 ml)
   anhydrous lanolin
¾ cup (177 ml) grapeseed
   or apricot kernel oil
1 teaspoon (5 ml) borax
1 tablespoon (15 ml)
   beeswax
1 tablespoon (15 ml) cocoa
   butter
15 drops essential oil of
   sandalwood or carrot
   seed

Good for: normal and dry skin
Use: daily or as desired
Prep time: approximately 40 minutes
Mix with: whisk
Store in: plastic squeeze bottle
Yields: approximately 8 applications
Special: Leaves skin very soft and smooth.
Can be used daily as a regular moisturizing
lotion.

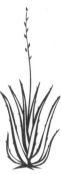

In a medium-sized saucepan over low heat or in a double boiler, combine the lanolin, oil (except essential oil), beeswax, and cocoa butter, and heat just until wax is melted. In another small saucepan, warm the aloe vera gel and herb tea. Slowly stir in the borax until dissolved. Remove both pans from heat. Slowly pour the borax mixture into the wax/oil mixture while stirring constantly with your whisk. Stir occasionally while it cools. When almost cool, add essential oil and stir again to mix. Store. Use approximately 3 tablespoons (44 ml) per use. Discard after 30 days. Does not provide sun protection.

SUNSCREEN BODY OIL

¼ cup (59 ml) anhydrous lanolin

¼ cup (59 ml) light sesame oil

4 teaspoons (20 ml) vitamin E oil

¼ cup (59 ml) sweet almond oil

⅓ (79 ml) cup aloe vera gel

15 drops essential oil of sandalwood or bitter almond

Good for: normal and dry skin; dark or tanned skin or when *minimal* sunscreen protection is desired

Use: before and during sun exposure

Prep time: approximately 10 minutes

Mix with: shake before use

Store in: plastic squeeze bottle

Yields: approximately 9 applications

Special: Makes a great after-bath skin softener.

Combine all ingredients in one or two squeeze bottles. Store the bottle you're not using in the refrigerator. Use approximately 2 tablespoons (30 ml) per use. Use unrefrigerated oil within 3 weeks or discard.

A note about sunscreens

I feel that the best nonchemical, highly effective sunscreens are the new titanium dioxide-based sunscreens. They can be used by all skin types, even sensitive, and are relatively sweat- and swim-proof. Origins (by Estée Lauder) is an excellent brand with many herbal extracts and my personal favorite.

SUNBURN RELIEF SUGGESTIONS

1. Add 2 cups (473 ml) apple cider vinegar to cool bath water and soak for 10 to 20 minutes.
2. Apply cold aloe vera gel directly to sunburn. Apply several times per day.
3. Apply cold, strong, regular tea directly to sunburn with soaked cotton pads. Apply several times per day.

FOR WOMEN ONLY: DOUCHES

Most dry form and premixed douches are chemical-based and can strip the natural protective pH of the vagina. As an alternative, the following recipes are very gentle. Keep in mind that these douches are not intended as a medical treatment but rather a cosmetic one. See your doctor if symptoms persist.

If you have any allergies related to plants, be sure to perform the patch test as described on page 33 before using either of these recipes.

VAGINITIS RELIEF

2 quarts (1.9 litres) luke-
   warm water
¼ cup (59 ml) apple cider
   vinegar *or* 10 drops
   essential oil of tea tree

Good for: external itching and burning; cleans excess vaginal discharge

Use: one to two times per week. Do not use more often than this.

Prep time: approximately 2 minutes

Yields: 1 treatment

Special: Leaves a clean, fresh feeling.

Combine ingredients in a 2-quart (2 litres) douche bag and proceed as usual. See your doctor if symptoms persist.

FRESHENING DOUCHE

2 quarts (1.9 litres) water
2 tablespoons (30 ml)
   peppermint, rosemary,
   or yarrow

Good for: general cleansing and freshening

Use: one time per week

Prep time: approximately 2 hours

Yields: 1 treatment

Boil water and remove from heat. Add herb, cover, and steep for about 2 hours. Strain and pour into douche bag. Proceed as usual.

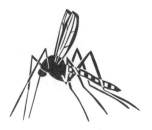

INSECT REPELLENT

This insect repellent recipe is a natural alternative to chemical sprays. It works best on days when the mosquitoes are only slightly to moderately hungry. If they're voracious, a stronger concoction will have to be sought.

INSECT REPELLENT

2 cups (473 ml) witch hazel

1½ teaspoons (7.5 ml) essential oil of citronella or lemongrass

1 tablespoon (15 ml) apple cider vinegar

Good for: all skin types

Use: as needed

Prep time: 3 to 5 minutes

Mix with: shake before use

Store in: spritzer

Yields: approximately 50 applications for entire body

Special: Has a light, fresh fragrance.

Combine all ingredients in a 16-ounce (480 ml) spray bottle or two 8-ounce (240 ml) bottles. Shake vigorously. Requires no refrigeration. Apply liberally as needed. Keep away from eyes, nose, and mouth.

APPENDIX A: INGREDIENT SOURCES

Aphrodisia
282 Bleecker Street
New York, NY 10014
(212) 989-6440
Extensive line of herbal care products, including essential oils, herbs, spices, natural soaps, bath salts, base oils, and additive-free green, red, yellow, rose, and white clay

Aroma Vera
5901 Rodeo Road
Los Angeles, CA 90016-4312
(800) 669-9514
Essential oils, natural skin care and bath products, hair care, and books

Aura Cacia
P.O. Box 399
Weaverville, CA 96093
(800) 437-3301
Essential and base oils for bath and massage

Avena Botanicals
20 Mill Street
Rockland, ME 04841
(207) 594-0694
Herbal products, herbs, and essential oils. Catalog $2.00.

Costello Imports
561 Broadway
Sonoma, CA 95476
(800) 388-7273
Additive-free powdered green, red, yellow, rose, and white clay. The green clay is also available in a wet form.

Indiana Botanic Gardens, Inc.
3401 West Thirty-Seventh Avenue
Hobart, IN 46342
(219) 947-4040
Herbs, essential oils, resins, and herbal preparations

Lavender Lane
6715 Donerail Drive
Sacramento, CA 95842
(916) 334-4400
Essential, fragrance, and base oils for bath and massage. Also, has a wonderful variety of bottles and jars for storing your cosmetic creations. Good prices!

Logee's Greenhouse
North Street
Danielson, CT 06239
Offer rare, fragrant flowering and herbal plants. Send $3.00 (refundable) for catalog.

Lorann Oils
4518 Aurelius Road
P.O. Box 22009
Lansing, MI 48909-2009
(800) 248-1302 outside Michigan
(800) 862-8620 within Michigan
Essential, flavor, and base oils and a few cosmetic ingredients

Mountain Rose
Box 2000
Redway, CA 95560
(800) 879-3337
Herbs, teas, essential oils, herbal body care products, and herbalist supplies

Nature's Herb Co.
1010 Forty-Sixth Street
Emeryville, CA 94608
(415) 601-0700
Herbs, potpourri ingredients, essential oils, and other kitchen cosmetic supplies

Penn Herb Co., Ltd.
603 North Second Street
Philadelphia, PA 19123-3098
(800) 523-9971
Established in 1924, this company carries essential oils, herbal extracts, natural foods, and almost every herb you can imagine. They also have an excellent assortment of herb and health books.

Renaissance Acres
4450 Valentine
Whitmore Lake, MI 48189
Sell organically raised herb plants,
seeds, and dried herbs. Send $2.00 for
catalog.

Sappo Hill Soapworks
654 Tolman Creek Road
Ashland, OR 97520
(503) 482-4485
All-natural glycerin creme, and oatmeal
and cornmeal soaps. Their glycerin
soaps can be grated and used as a base
to make your own herbal soap balls.

The Original Swiss Aromatics
P.O. Box 6842
28 Paul Drive, Suite F
San Rafael, CA 94903
(415) 459-3998
Essential and base oils, perfumes, and
natural cosmetics

The Preferred Source
3637 West Alabama, Suite 160
Houston, TX 77027
(713) 622-2190
Essential oils

Walnut Acres Farm
Penns Creek, PA 17862
(800) 433-3998
Organically grown, natural foods direct
from the farm. Hundreds of fresh,
delicious foods on the premises, ready
for shipment. I find their catalog to be
one of the best sources for organic
grains and raw, dried fruits and nuts.

Weleda, Inc.
P. O. Box 249
Congers, NY 10920
(914) 268-8572
(800) 241-1030
Natural cosmetics, some essential oils,
herbs, and tea

APPENDIX B: SUGGESTED READING

Herb Books

Bremness, Lesley. **Herbs.**
The Reader's Digest Association, Inc.

Buchman, Dian Dincin.
**The Complete Herbal Guide to
Natural Health and Beauty.**
Doubleday & Co., Inc.

Garland, Sarah. **The Complete Book
of Herbs and Spices.**
The Viking Press

Jacobs, Betty E.M. **Growing & Using
Herbs Successfully.**
Storey Communications, Inc.

Kloss, Jethro. **Back to Eden.**
Woodbridge Press Publishing Co.

Lust, John, N.D., D.B.M.
The Herb Book.
Bantam Books

**Rodale's Illustrated Encyclopedia
of Herbs.**
Rodale Press.

Malcolm, Stuart. **The Encyclopedia
of Herbs & Herbalism.**
Cresent Books

Weiss, Gaea and Shandor.
Growing & Using the Healing Herbs.
Rodale Press

Worwood, Valerie Ann.
**The Complete Book of Essential
Oils and Aromatherapy.**
New World Library

APPENDIX C: PERIODICALS & NEWSLETTERS

The Herbal Connection
P.O. Box 245
Silver Springs, PA 17575
A bi-monthly newsletter for herbal
enthusiasts and herb business owners.

HerbalGram
P.O. Box 201660
Austin, TX 78720
(512) 331-8868
A quarterly journal of the American
Botanical Council and Herb Research
Foundation

The Herb Companion
201 East Fourth Street
Loveland, CO 80537
A bi-monthly magazine for the herb
enthusiast.

The Herb Quarterly
P.O. Box 689
San Anselmo, CA 94960
(415) 455-9540

The Herb Society of America
9019 Kirtland-Charton Road
Mentor, OH 44060
Send a self-addressed, stamped envelope and $.50 for their latest list of
herb publications.

Vegetarian Times
P.O. Box 570
Oak Park, IL 60303
(708) 848-8100
A monthly magazine covering diet and
nutrition with frequent contributions
by practicing herbalists

APPENDIX D: HERBAL CORRESPONDENCE COURSES

Aromatherapy Seminars
1830 South Robertson Boulevard
Suite 203
Los Angeles, CA 90035
(800) 677-2368

Emerson College of Herbology, Ltd.
Dept. A
582 Cummer Avenue
Willowdale, ON M2K 2M4
(416) 733-2512

Pacific Institute of Aromatherapy
P.O. Box 6723
San Rafael, CA 94903
(415) 479-9121

**Rocky Mountain Center for
Botanical Studies**
P.O. Box 19254
Boulder, CO 80308-2254
(303) 442-6861

The Science and Art of Herbology
By Rosemary Gladstar
Send $20.00 for Lesson 1 and informa-
tion to: SAGE, P.O. Box 420, E. Barre, VT
05649
(802) 479-9825

APPENDIX E: NUTRITION & DIET BOOKS

Airola, Paavo, Ph.D. **How To Get Well.** Health Plus Publishers
Contains detailed section on dry brushing

Bates, Dorothy R. **The TVP Cookbook.** The Book Publishing Company

Colbin, Annemarie. **The Book of Whole Meals.** Ballantine Books

Diamond, Harvey and Diamond, Marilyn. **Fit for Life.** Warner Books, Inc.

Diamond, Harvey and Diamond, Marilyn. **Living Healthy.** Warner Books, Inc.

Garrison, Robert H., Jr., M.A., R.Ph., and Somer, Elizabeth, M.A., R.D. **The Nutrition Desk Reference.** Keats Publishing, Inc.

McDougall, John A., M.D. and McDougall, Mary, L.P.N. **The McDougall Plan.** New Century Publishers, Inc.

McDougall, John A., M.D. and McDougall, Mary, L.P.N. **The McDougall Program.** Penguin Books

Robbins, John. **Diet For A New America.** Stillpoint Publishing

Soltanoff, Jack D.C. **Natural Healing.** Warner Books, Inc.

BIBLIOGRAPHY

Gerson, Joel. *Standard Textbook for Professional Estheticians.* Bronx, NY: MILADY Publishing Corp., 1986.

Kloss, Jethro. *Back to Eden.* Santa Barbara, CA: Woodbridge Press Publishing Co., 1939.

Lust, John B., N.D., D.B.M. *The Herb Book.* New York, NY: Bantam Books, 1974.

McCarter, Drs. Robert and Elizabeth. *Nutrition and the Skin. The Life Science Health System, Part XII:* Natural Hygiene: A Better Way of Living, Lesson 61. Austin, TX: College of Life Science, 1983.

Sarfati, Lydia. *Repechage Professional Skin Care Manual.* New York, NY: Sarkli-Repechage, Ltd., 1984.

Soltanoff, Jack, D.C. *Natural Healing.* New York, NY: Warner Books, Inc., 1988.

INDEX